Department of Health and Social Security

Lead and Health

The Report of a DHSS Working Party on Lead in the Environment

[1980]

London—Her Majesty's Stationery Office

ISBN 0 11 320728 X

Foreword

1 This report by Professor Lawther's Working Party is the latest in a series of reviews of this subject both here and abroad. I believe that it is a valuable and timely addition to international work on environmental exposure to lead. I particularly welcome the breadth of the Working Party's approach, and its attempt to evaluate the significance of all the various ways in which people may be exposed to environmental lead; this provides an essential basis for considering priorities for action. On behalf of HM Government I should therefore like to thank Professor Lawther and the members of his Working Party for producing such an excellent and comprehensive report.

2 Since publication in 1974 of the interdepartmental report 'Lead in the Environment and its Significance to Man', it has been the policy of successive Governments that people's exposure to lead pollution should be contained and wherever practicable reduced, particularly in those circumstances where people are most exposed to risk. Action has been and is being taken on a range of sources of environmental lead.

3 The Working Party recommends further action in a number of fields. I and my colleagues will consider these recommendations in the light of the evidence assembled by the Working Party and of the practical and economic factors that must be taken into account. We shall undertake this process with all practicable speed.

4 It gives me particular pleasure to be able to welcome the report since a distinguished ancestor of mine, Robert Christison MD, Professor of Materia Medica in the University of Edinburgh carried out some pioneering research on lead pollution in the 1830s and 1840s.

PATRICK JENKIN,
Secretary of State for Social Services.

Contents

Note on Terms

Kg	kilogram, one thousand grams
g	gram
mg	milligram, one thousandth of a gram
μg	microgram, one millionth of a gram
mg/kg	milligrams per kilogram, equivalent to parts per million
μg/kg	micrograms per kilogram, equivalent to parts per thousand million
l	litre
dl	decilitre, one tenth of a litre or 100 millilitres
ml	millilitre, one thousandth of a litre
m	metre
Km	kilometre, one thousand metres
mm	millimetre, one thousandth of a metre
μm	micron, one millionth of a metre
mol	molecular weight
μ mol	one millionth of the molecular weight
μg/dl	one microgram per decilitre or one microgram per 100 ml
μ mol/l	one millionth of the molecular weight per litre (SI units) For lead 1μg/dl is the same as 0.048 μ mol/litre or 21 μg/dl is approximately equal to 1μ mol/litre
d	day
Cal	calorie
K cal	kilo calorie, one thousand calories

1 Introduction

1 Lead and its compounds are potentially toxic; the element has no known physiological functions; it is widely distributed in nature and as a result of man's activities. The gross effects which it can have on health have been recognised for many years and there are now relatively few cases of frank lead poisoning in this country. However, reports in recent years have suggested that there could be ill effects from exposure to lead in amounts which are too small to cause the classical signs and symptoms of lead poisoning.

2 The Department of Health & Social Security Working Party on Lead was established in November 1978. The terms of reference were 'To review the overall effects on health of environmental lead from all sources and, in particular, its effects on the health and development of children and to assess the contribution lead in petrol makes to the body burden'. Independent experts actively engaged in the fields of clinical paediatrics, pathology, child psychiatry, psychology, epidemiology and the environmental sciences were appointed. Members of the Working Party are listed in Appendix 1. Owing to the complexity of the problem put to the Working Party scrutiny of a wide range of studies was essential and a bibliography of nearly 3,000 publications was compiled. A list of the scientific papers to which special attention was given is shown in Appendix 4 and a copy of the full list of references has been deposited at the British Library.

3 Man has always absorbed some lead from his natural environment, although this contribution is usually small in comparison with that derived from lead liberated by his own activities. Food may contain small amounts of lead from canning processes, contact with glazed containers and deposition from polluted air. Major contributions to the body burden may be made in some areas by lead water pipes and lead-lined storage tanks; lead compounds have been commonly used in paints and primers in the past and the risk to young children who chew old painted surfaces is well known. The production and industrial use of lead may also give rise to much dust and fumes within factories and their immediate environment. All these potential

sources of exposure to lead are well known and a variety of measures including regulations have done much to reduce the risks in the UK.

4 Among the many sources of lead, special concern has been voiced about pollution of the air by petrol engines using fuel to which alkyl lead compounds have been added to improve the octane rating. This practice began over 50 years ago and, although the lead content of petrol has been reduced in recent years, the increase in the use of this fuel has led to it becoming the major contributor of lead in the air in this and most other developed countries. Airborne lead may be taken in not only directly by inhalation but also by ingestion, through the contamination of food and dust. It is important however, to consider airborne lead in the context of lead from all sources; its significance can be assessed only when the contributions from food, water, air and the various adventitious sources have been determined.

5 The clinical manifestations of substantial quantities of lead are well known and much work has been published on the toxic effects which amongst adults usually result from occupational exposure. The occurrence of clinical lead poisoning and its sequelae in children, particularly following the ingestion of lead-based paint by those with pica (defined in paragraph 142) is also well documented. It is well known that elevated blood lead concentrations can be seen in children with this habit even in the absence of symptoms.

6 The main question with which we were concerned was the possibility that more subtle adverse effects on health and development may result from the chronic absorption of lead in smaller quantities than those known to give symptoms or signs and hitherto thought to be without effect. During recent years many reports, notably from the USA, have suggested that lead might interfere with mental development or cause behavioural disorders in children. The evidence though suggestive is equivocal and difficult to assess.

7 The report deals in sequence with the several sources of lead in the environment, with the relative importance of each of these to the uptake of lead and with the neuropsychological effects of lead on children. Following a general discussion the report concludes with recommendations for action and research. We have not reported on the extensive literature which we have considered on clinical lead poisoning, or on experimental work in animals and biochemical mechanisms. Such work throws light on the ways in which relatively small amounts of lead might have an effect but it does not determine whether they have effects of medical or social significance. We have therefore concentrated our attention on the evidence from human populations, which has been widely regarded as critical to this issue.

8 During the course of 1979 the Department of the Environment has co-ordinated a number of blood lead surveys in different areas of the country in fulfilment of an EEC Directive on the Biological Screening of the Population for Lead (CEC, 1977). The results of the surveys have extended our knowledge of the distribution of blood lead concentrations among the general adult population and among children who may be exposed to above average concentrations of lead. The provisional results available at the time of completion of the report are reproduced in Appendix 2.

9 We wish to record our indebtedness to many Government Departments for the unflagging help given in the provision of information, to outside experts who gave us special advice on particular issues, and to many others who supplied information and opinions. We would like to express particular gratitude to the Secretariat for its unstinted labour and support, without which we would have been unable to complete this work in little more than a year.

2 Lead From Food

10 The evidence which is available on human exposure to lead indicates that, for the population as a whole, the diet is the most important route of exposure. The majority of the environmental sources of lead contribute directly or indirectly.

Sources of Lead in Food

11 Some of the lead in food comes from the soil as a result of the natural weathering of lead-rich ores and minerals. Some is derived from human activities, in 3 main ways:

a. contamination of canned food by lead solder used in making cans;

b. contamination by lead plumbing systems of tap water used in cooking;

c. contamination of soil, crops and food by lead in air and dust.

The contribution of each of these sources to the intake of lead is discussed in paragraphs 26-31.

Surveys of Lead Intake

12 Estimates of the amount of lead consumed in the diet are difficult to obtain. Dietary habits vary widely; the long-term intake, which determines any effects on health, can only be estimated approximately. There are two ways in which it is practicable to estimate the amount of lead which is consumed. Firstly, lead can be measured in artificial diets made up specially to represent an average national diet (total diet studies). Secondly, it can be measured by analysis of a representative proportion of the food actually consumed by individuals who are selected for study (individual diet studies). Both of these approaches have been adopted by the Ministry of Agriculture, Fisheries and Food (MAFF).

Total Diet Studies

13 Each year since 1974, MAFF has estimated the average intake of lead by means of a total diet study. These studies are based on information obtained from the National Food Survey and the National Household Expenditure Survey on the average amounts of food purchased by households in this country. An estimate of the average amount of foods which are consumed can be derived from this information by allowing for the food which is bought but not eaten. Colleges of Domestic Science in various parts of the United Kingdom purchase locally the food necessary to make up a standard diet based on these statistics and then prepare and cook the food as appropriate. The concentration of lead in each of various groups of food is analysed so that the average daily intake of lead of the population can be calculated.

14 Since 1974 a total of 113 such diets have been analysed, made up from foods purchased throughout the UK. The calculated intake of lead per head has varied between 55 and 366 µg/day with a mean of 113 µg/day.

15 It is important to note that when diets are analysed many individual food groups contain lead at or below the limit of detection by the method of analysis. In such cases it is assumed that lead is present at the lower limit of detection. The intakes of lead are therefore probably overestimated.

16 Although total diet studies do not take into account variations in dietary habit, it has been found that the concentration of lead in most of the food groups is similar. Consequently a personal preference for any one type of food is not liable to affect exposure to lead substantially. The intake of lead is likely to be more related to the total amount of food consumed.

Table 1 Energy requirements and corresponding dietary lead intakes of adult males and children

	Energy requirements (Kcal)	Lead intake (µg/day)
UK Average	2,200(a)	113
Adult male	2,850(b)	146
Children (2 years)	1,350	70
(3–4 years)	1,530	80

(a) Associated with food consumption of 1.34 kg per day.
(b) Requirement of a 15–17 year old or a moderately active male.

17 The lead intakes quoted above are averages for the population of the UK as a whole. It is possible to estimate average intakes for sub-groups of the population, such as adult males or children, by adjusting for their average energy requirements compared with the average energy requirements of the total population. The results of such calculations are set out in Table 1 and show an average lead intake of 146 μg/day for adult males and of 70 to 80 μg/day for 2-4 year old children. For this purpose it is assumed that the children consume the same type of diet as adults.

Individual Diet Studies

18 In these studies identical duplicates of all food eaten by the individual whose diet is being studied are set aside after cooking. Milk and both alcoholic and non-alcoholic beverages are excluded. These 'duplicate diets' are then blended and analysed for lead. Practical constraints limit the number and duration of these studies but MAFF have analysed duplicate samples of the food intake of adults and young infants for one week in a few such studies in various localities.

19 A total of 195 weekly diets of selected adults have been analysed. The dietary intakes were found to range between 21 and 330 microgrammes per day with an average of 75 microgrammes per day. (MAFF, unpublished data).

Individual Diet Studies in Infants

20 The dietary intake of lead of infants up to 4 months of age has been measured in a recent duplicate diet study. Three hundred infants were selected at random from the birth registers in each of six towns in England and Wales and their weekly diets analysed. The results for bottle-fed babies are summarised in Table 2. Since infant diets are restricted, these intakes are likely to be representative of the level of exposure of infants up to the age of 6 months or until feeding with solids begins.

Table 2 Dietary lead intakes of bottle-fed infants

Intake	Range	Mean
Intake μg per day	6–99	17
Intake μg/kg bodyweight per day	0.7–30	3

21 The wide range of these results is largely explained by the very different levels of water lead found in the study. The concentrations of lead found in dehydrated infant food ranges from 10–300 µg/kg with a mean level of 150 µg/kg (MAFF, 1975). Since the proportion of liquids to solids in the prepared feed is 8:1 the lead present in the solids would provide a large proportion of intake only if lead in tap water was less than 20 µg/1; it would never be an important source nor could it explain the higher intakes found within this study. The contribution that may be made by lead-containing water to lead intakes in artifically fed infants is dealt with in Chapter 3.

22 In comparison with these findings recent work indicates that the concentrations of lead found in breast milk are about 10% of the blood lead level of the mother (M R Moore, unpublished data). It is unlikely, therefore, that breast milk contains lead in excess of 3 µg/litre among women in the general population, equivalent to an intake of 0.45 µg/kg body weight per day in infants.

Total Intake of Lead – Conclusions

23 The results of the diet studies give sound estimates of the exposure of individuals or populations at a given time. The analysis of a single diet sample, however, does not necessarily represent long-term intake and the results of the individual diet studies (paragraph 19) probably exaggerate the range of long-term lead intakes.

24 On the basis of the dietary studies carried out so far, it is probable that the great majority of the long-term average dietary intakes of lead of individual adults are within the range 70 to 150 µg/day; they are probably closer to the lower figure for the reasons stated in paragraph 15. These figures will be used in Chapter 6 in estimating the relative contribution of food to the total intake of lead.

Official Guidelines for Dietary Lead

25 The Joint Food and Agriculture World Health Organisation (FAO/WHO) Expert Committee on Food Additives has suggested a provisional tolerable weekly intake of 3.0 mg of lead for adults (FAO/WHO, 1972), equivalent to about 430 µg/day. This is well above the dietary intakes found in the United Kingdom as described above. The maximum amount of lead in foods offered for sale in the United Kingdom has been subject to control for some

time. The Lead in Food Regulations were revised in 1979 and provide a maximum permitted general limit of the lead content in food of 1.0 mg/kg (=1 ppm). They also impose individual limits on a list of specified foods and limit the lead content of foods specially prepared for young infants to 0.2 mg/kg unless such foods are sold in a dried, dehydrated or concentrated form, in which case the specified limit is 1.0 mg/kg. These regulations specify the maximum quantity of lead that an individual food may contain but the amount normally found is considerably lower. Thus the limits do not reflect the normal dietary intake.

The Contribution of Individual Sources of Lead to Dietary Intake

Canned Food

26 Solder used in the manufacture of cans is the only recognised source of contamination of food by lead during processing. Data on the production of canned food in the UK, adjusted for imports and exports, allow an estimate to be made of the average consumption per head of individual types of canned food. Most canned food, excluding beverages, which is sold in the UK is confined to a few products; these account for annual sales of 1.3 million tonnes. From a knowledge of the mean lead levels in these products, it is calculated that they contribute approximately 15% of the total daily dietary intake of lead. A wide range of other canned food (0.3 million tonnes) is sold but there are insufficient data on lead content to give a more accurate assessment of intake from this source. In general canned beverages are not an important source of lead and the available information suggests that the average concentrations of lead in such products are less than 20 µg/kg (MAFF, 1975).

27 A recent total diet study (MAFF, unpublished) compared the amount of lead in diets containing an average proportion of canned food with that in equivalent diets containing only non-canned food. The study indicated that the use of canned food is likely to contribute about 15% to the total dietary intake of lead. This estimate agrees with that quoted in paragraph 26.

28 The maximum concentration of lead which is permitted in prepared foods specifically intended for babies or young children is 200 µg/kg. (Lead in Food Regulations, 1979). This regulation has meant that manufacturers have had to use pure tin solder for canning infant foods. As a result no more lead is found in these foods than that which is present in the raw materials from which they are made.

29 The contribution to lead in food which is made by any lead in the tap water used in cooking has been studied by MAFF (Unpublished). Samples of hard and soft water containing different amounts of lead were obtained by leaving the waters in contact with lead piping for a long time and then diluting them with distilled water. Most water for cooking is used in the preparation of green and root vegetables; each of these foods was therefore cooked in the different samples of water and the concentrations of lead in the cooked food was measured. From a knowledge of the intake of lead from other foods in the average diet (paragraph 13) the contribution made to lead in food by cooking with water at different concentrations of lead were calculated. The results are shown in Table 3.

Table 3 Contribution of lead in cooking water to total intake of lead from food

Type of water	Lead in water μg/l	Daily intake of lead from food μg/day				Lead from cooking water as a % of total
		Vegetables	Other food	Total	From cooking water	
(1)	(2)	(3)	(4)	(5)	(6)	(7)
Hard	520	130	} 64	194	107	55
	265	74		138	51	37
	135	46		110	23	21
	0*	23		87	0	0
Soft	250	67	} 64	131	52	40
	105	28		92	13	14
	55	23		87	8	9
	0*	15		79	0	0

NOTES

*Below limit of detection (distilled water).

COL. 3. Lead from root and green vegetables cooked in each sample of water.

COL. 4. Lead from other foods (as determined by the 1978 total diet study).

COL. 5. Col. 3 + Col. 4.

COL. 6. Col. 3 less amount of lead in vegetables cooked in distilled water (23 and 15 μg/d).

COL. 7. Col. 6 as a % of Col. 5.

30 Column 7 of Table 3 shows the proportion of lead in food which would come from water containing different amounts of lead. The proportion is likely to be more than 15% when lead in water exceeds 100 μg/l, whereas it

would be only about 3% with concentrations about the relatively common value of 20 µg/l. People who eat large amounts of cooked vegetables or other foods made up with or cooked in water, could have higher intakes from this source. No account is taken here of the effect of lead in water on the intake from beverages made in the home (which are considered in Chapter 3).

The Contribution of Lead in Air and Dust

31 Some part of the lead in food is derived from car exhaust emissions, the use of fossil fuels, lead smelting, etc. (See Chapter 4). Airborne lead from these sources may be deposited directly on food and crops; it may permanently contaminate soil and be taken up by plants (although on the basis of existing information this effect is likely to be small), or it may contaminate dust which may then be blown onto food and crops. In particular, fruit and vegetables grown near busy roads and smelters are liable to be contaminated by airborne lead. However, the majority of these foods have a short growing season and are not heavily contaminated. In the case of leafy vegetables much of the deposited lead will be removed during preparation, washing and cooking, especially if the outer leaves are discarded. Crops grown near sources of airborne lead generally make only a small contribution to the diet and thus to the intake of lead.

Other Sources

32 The use of sewage sludge as fertiliser may also result in some contamination of crops by lead. Lead enters the sewers from industry, domestic discharges, or in run-off from roads. Lead arsenate has been a traditionally favoured insecticide but its use, for orchard fruits, is now extremely limited. No other agricultural or food processing activities involving a lead hazard have come to our attention.

3 Lead From Tap Water

33 Lead is rarely present in mains water. It is sometimes present in tap water, since it is liberated by certain types of 'plumbosolvent' water from any lead in domestic plumbing or the pipes which connect it to the mains.

34 The contribution of tap water to the total intake of lead depends on:

a. The amount of lead in tap water;

b. the amount of water consumed;

c. transfers of lead between food and water during cooking.

Amounts of Lead in Tap Water in Great Britain

35 Information on the concentrations of lead in water at the tap in Great Britain is available from the report 'Lead in Drinking Water—A Survey in Great Britain 1975-1976' (DOE, 1977). This elaborate and carefully designed survey was based on a random sample of more than 3,000 households and allowed statistically reliable estimates to be made of the number of households with different concentrations of lead in single samples of water at a given time in England, Scotland and Wales (but not in smaller geographical units). Two types of sample of water were taken from each household, both without preliminary flushing; one was a first draw sample and the other was taken at casual times in the day (daytime sample). The main results are given in Table 4 and are for daytime samples only since relatively little first draw water is consumed (Water Research Centre, in preparation). Concentrations in first draw samples were higher.

36 The report showed that, at the time of the survey, most households in Great Britain had little lead in their tap water but 10.3% had more than 50 µg/l in a single, unflushed, daytime sample and 4.3% had more than 100 µg/l. A few very high concentrations were recorded with one value greater than 1700 µg/l. The table shows that, on the basis of this recent evidence, high concentrations of lead in water are much more common in Scotland than in England or Wales.

Table 4 Lead in tap water in Great Britain

Lead concentration in daytime sample (μg/1)	Percentage of households			
	England	Scotland	Wales	Total
0– 9	66.0	46.4	70.5	64.5
10– 50	26.2	19.2	20.7	25.3
51–100	5.2	13.4	6.5	6.0
101–300	2.2	16.0	1.5	3.4
301 and above	0.4	5.0	0.8	0.9
Total	100.0	100.0	100.0	100.0

37 These figures may overestimate the proportion of people exposed to relatively high concentrations of lead in water for two reasons. Firstly, a substantial proportion of people run some water to waste or for other purposes before drawing it for consumption and the lead content is generally lower after flushing (Water Research Centre, unpublished; Thomas *et al*, 1979.) Secondly, local surveys have shown that there is marked variation in the concentration of lead in tap water within any household. Results based on single samples may therefore overestimate the proportion which would have high concentrations, if the value for each household were an average based on several samples. (On the other hand, such results *under*estimate the proportion of households with high concentrations of lead in water at *some* time.) A person's intake of lead over a period tends to reflect average concentrations and it is not possible to estimate intake, accurately, on the basis of single samples of tap water.

38 The amount of lead in a sample of tap water is primarily determined by the chemical characteristics of the water and the length of the lead piping through which it has run. Although it is widely known that soft, acid waters dissolve lead, the national survey showed that some harder waters also do so, although to a lesser extent. The factors which determine whether a hard water is plumbosolvent are at present not fully understood. Particularly high concentrations of lead are often found in places where the drinking water supply is drawn from the down pipe, in a lead plumbed house, especially if the roof tank is lead lined; this arrangement is common in Scotland, where at the same time soft acid waters predominate.

39 The concentration of lead in water is also influenced by the length of time the water has stood in the pipes. It also varies according to how far and how quickly the tap is turned and appears to be greater with the increase of temperature in summer (Water Research Centre, unpublished). The concen-

18

tration of lead can rise within hours when water stands in the pipes but flushing may achieve a substantial reduction in the lead content of water intended for consumption. Thomas *et al* (1979) showed that up to an eight-fold reduction can be achieved by flushing. Their results relate to exceptionally high initial concentrations but serve to suggest that, in many situations, otherwise unsuitable tap water might be made satisfactory by flushing; this will not be so where lead lined roof tanks are used. Water drawn from the hot tap may have a high lead content and is undesirable for cooking or to fill a kettle. This is true even in houses without lead plumbing since hot water is liable to leach lead from solder in copper tanks or piping.

Proposed Limit for Lead in Tap Water

40 An EEC Directive on the 'Quality of Water for Human Consumption' has been agreed, subject to some points of detail and is expected to specify a maximum of 50 µg/l for lead in water in non-lead plumbed houses. It is also expected to state that, where lead pipes are present, the lead content *should* not exceed 50 µg/l in a sample taken after flushing but to require that, 'if a sample is taken directly or after flushing and the lead content either frequently or to an appreciable extent exceeds 100 µg/l, suitable measures *must* be taken to reduce exposure to lead on the part of the consumer'.

41 The requirement concerning households with lead pipes may be regarded as specifying that it is the *average* from several samples of water as it is consumed in any household which should not exceed 100 µg/l; in that case some individual values may be above 100 µg/l simply because of the variability of water lead in any household.

42 The Directive is expected to allow 5 years for compliance, with a longer period in exceptional cases, provided that an action programme and a timetable for compliance are accepted by the European Commission.

Action in Great Britain to Reduce Lead in Tap Water

43 Much has already been done by the British water industry. Surveys have been carried out in many parts of the country to identify the general areas where action is needed. Some sources of plumbosolvent water have been replaced and a number of schemes to reduce plumbosolvency by chemical treatment have been introduced or are planned. Substantial reductions in lead concentrations have already been achieved by chemical treatment in

19

places such as Glasgow. Lead plumbing is commonly replaced when housing is modernised and, occasionally, to deal with isolated examples of consistently high water lead levels in houses. Thomas *et al* (1979) have described the effects of pipe replacement in a housing estate where water lead concentrations had been exceptionally high; the results are discussed in paragraph 103. Further action is planned by the industry and much supporting research is being done by the Water Research Centre and the water undertakings.

44 It is hoped that chemical treatment will generally suffice to reduce water lead to the desired concentrations. It is effective in many circumstances but there are technical difficulties (in particular with some harder plumbosolvent waters) and, in spite of intensive research, it cannot be assumed that these will be fully overcome. We have been told that the early replacement of lead pipes on a very large scale is not a practicable solution due to costs and the extent of the requirement for trained labour and suitable material. Other methods such as pipe-lining are being investigated but none looks promising at present.

Future Concentrations of Lead in Water

45 It is too early to predict the future pattern of water lead concentrations or the time which will be taken to complete the programme of action. The reduction in lead levels will be greatest in soft, acidic waters where present concentrations are highest. In the case of plumbosolvent waters of high alkalinity it is too early to predict what can be achieved by water treatment; current lead concentrations in these waters do not, however, reach the high values which may be found in acidic waters. There is thought to be a good chance that chemical treatment will succeed in reducing the *average* concentration of lead in unflushed daytime samples of water to below 100 µg/l, except in houses where lead lined roof tanks are in use. If not, it should be practicable to deal with the remaining cases by such means as flushing or some measure of pipe replacement. Either lead lined tanks will have to be replaced or lined, or the contamination of drinking water minimized by supplying the kitchen tap from the rising main.

46 It will take several years to identify all the affected localities and to develop and install treatment although much has already been done in the most seriously affected areas. It should therefore be considered whether any interim measures are possible and desirable.

The Consumption of Drinking Water

47 A Water Research Centre survey (report in preparation) has provided information on the amount of drinking water consumed by people in various age groups in Great Britain. The results are given in Table 5. The average adult consumes about 1 litre a day but consumption may be as high as 2¾ litres per day. The amount consumed includes all tap water, whether drunk at home or elsewhere, and beverages made from tap water, but not commercial drinks or water used in cooking.

Table 5 Total consumption of tap water at home and elsewhere
GB both sexes

Age Years	Total consumption of tap water litres/head/day		
	Minimum†	Mean	Maximum‡
1– 3	*	0.50	*
3–14	0.04	0.57	1.54
15+	0.21	1.07	2.73

*Sample size too small for reliable estimate.
†Under 1% in each age group consume less than the minimum value.
‡Under 1% in each age group consume more than the maximum value.

48 Artificially fed infants drink approximately 0.15 1/kg/day and may take more in hot weather. They are particularly likely to be affected by the undesirable habit of filling kettles from the hot tap.

Transfer of Lead from Water During Cooking

49 Lead is transferred from lead-containing tap water to some foods during preparation and cooking. Research to determine the extent of the transfer is described in paragraphs 29 and 30. It indicates that the net effect, for the average adult eating a typical British diet, is roughly equivalent to drinking an extra 0.18 1 a day of the same tap water. (This estimate is obtained by dividing the figures in column 6 of Table 3 by the equivalent figures in column 2 and averaging and rounding the results.)

Total Intake of Lead from Water

50 Using the figures in Table 5 for water consumption and a range of lead concentrations, total intakes of lead from water by adults who consume an average amount of water, adults who consume the maximum amount and artificially fed infants have been calculated for the Working Party. The results are set out in Table 6; the figures include an allowance for lead transferred from water to food during cooking. It should be noted that some of the diets in the total diet studies discussed in paragraphs 13 to 17 were prepared with lead-containing water so that there is an element of double counting between the estimates of intake from food in that section of the report and from water in this. The figures for lead concentrations refer to the average concentrations for households.

Table 6 Daily lead intake from tap water

Daily consumption including allowance for cooking	Average concentration of lead in water (line a) Estimated daily intake of lead (lines b, c & d)								
	50		100		150		200		a
	μg/d	μg/kg/d*	μg/d	μg/kg/d*	μg/d	μg/kg/d*	μg/d	μg/kg/d*	
(1)	(2)	(3)	(4)	(5)	(6)	(7)	(8)	(9)	
Average for adult 1.25 l/day	62	1.0	125	2.0	188	3.0	250	4.0	b
Maximum for adult 2.9 l/day	145	2.3	290	4.6	435	7.0	580	9.3	c
Artificially fed infants 0.15 l/kg body weight/day	—	7.5	—	15.0	—	22.5	—	30.0	d

*For adults approximate values based upon average body weight.

51 Columns 2 and 3 of Table 6 illustrate intakes of lead from water which are, and are likely to continue to be, not uncommon. In Chapter 6 (paragraph 102) they will be taken as the upper limit of exposure to lead from water in cities not recognised as having a severe water lead problem.

52 Columns 4 and 5 show intakes of people consuming water which just complies with the EEC limit for lead plumbed houses. It is expected that all intakes will be below these levels when the national programme, based largely on chemical treatment, has been completed. The majority of people who will still have some lead in their tap water will have intakes which are substantially below these levels but these figures indicate that it will be possible for a small number of adults to have intakes approaching 300 μg/d until all lead plumbing is replaced. The proportion with intakes of this order will depend on the extent to which action is taken beyond that necessary to comply with the EEC Directive, but it will probably not be feasible to avoid such intakes altogether.

53 The intakes indicated in the last four columns may still be seen for some years in certain areas, until the national programme is completed. It is expected that, in the near future, substantially higher intakes than those illustrated here will no longer be encountered as a result of action now being taken or proposed in the worst affected areas.

4 Lead From Air

54 Lead occurs naturally throughout the world and is found in soils, in the oceans and in the air. Natural mobilisation by weathering of mineral deposits and gaseous emissions by volcanic activity are estimated to release about 210,000 tonnes of lead into the global environment each year (Goldberg and Gross, 1971). However, the concentration of lead in air due to natural sources is very low. In most developed parts of the world emissions from human activities in the winning, processing, and utilisation of lead provide the main contribution to airborne lead.

Major Sources of Lead in Air

55 Lead found as a component of the particulate matter in air results primarily from the combustion of lead-containing petrol and from certain industrial processes and to a lesser extent from the combustion of coal, and weathering of paints. The chemical and physical form of the lead varies widely according to the source. Much of the lead emitted from cars and from industrial processes after the waste gases have been cleaned is fine enough to remain airborne for long periods and is within the respirable size range. These small particles are widely dispersed and lead resulting from man's activities has been detected at the polar regions. Coarse particles are generally deposited close to their source and may contribute appreciably to the lead content of dust. The short period concentration of lead found in the atmosphere close to sources is likely to vary considerably as the source strength and factors affecting dispersion change. However, as it takes the human body some time (weeks or months) to come to equilibrium with intake and excretion of lead, it is normal to express the concentration of lead in air as a long-term mean, for example a 3-monthly or annual mean. The variation in concentration between such periods is much less than is found between short-term averages.

Lead in Petrol

56 In 1978, 10,300 tonnes of lead as organic lead compounds were added to the 18 million tonnes of petrol used in the United Kingdom. Some 7,000

tonnes of this lead are emitted, mostly as fine particulates, with the exhaust gases from petrol-engined vehicles, along with many other pollutants, including approximately 7½ million tonnes of carbon monoxide, 360,000 tonnes of hydrocarbons and 300,000 tonnes of oxides of nitrogen (DOE, 1979). Because of its wide dispersion only a minute proportion of the total lead emitted is liable to find its way directly into human beings. The particulate lead is mainly in the form of halides produced by reactions with the scavengers that are also added to petrol, but in the atmosphere these halides are converted gradually into oxides, carbonates and sulphates. The lead compounds emitted from petrol engines are commonly present in complex aggregates together with carbonaceous material and in this form they may be less available to man than if they were present in simpler form (Lawther *et al*, 1973). Some organic lead enters the atmosphere from the evaporation of petrol, and to a minor extent as unburned compounds in the exhaust. This gaseous component normally represents only a very small proportion of the total lead in the general urban atmosphere (Harrison and Perry, 1977; Rohbock *et al*, 1980).

57 The concentrations of airborne lead resulting from the use of leaded petrol depend on factors such as traffic density, traffic speed, weather conditions and local topography, and they can be high in or very close to busy roads. Annual mean concentrations of more than 12 $\mu g/m^3$ were measured at the central reservation of the M4 in 1974 and 1975 (Colwill, 1979, personal communication). Values for recent years at this site have fallen to about 9 $\mu g/m^3$ reflecting, among other factors, the changes in the lead content of petrol over the period. Annual mean concentrations measured in busy urban roads are usually within the range 2 to 6 $\mu g/m^3$. Mean concentrations over shorter periods, or those based on samples collected during daytime periods only, may be 2 or 3 times higher. Some typical values of roadside measurements are given in Table 7a (page 26). Also included are recent figures obtained near the M4 at Hillingdon and the North Circular Road at Neasden where corresponding blood lead values were measured under the EEC programme of blood lead surveillance. (See Appendix 2). The relatively high values, approaching 6 $\mu g/m^3$, for Heath Street, Hampstead, which are included in Table 7a were obtained at a first-floor flat facing directly onto a narrow street, on a hill, with much slow-moving private car traffic throughout the day. This combination of circumstances results in higher values than are found either in a busier central area, eg Fleet Street, where a large proportion of the traffic is diesel-engined, or close to motorways, where the more open situation and rapid movement aids dispersion.

58 The concentration of airborne lead decreases rapidly with distance away from roads; a graph illustrating this (Figure 1) suggests that concentrations

fall to about 20% of their kerbside value at a distance of 50m. At greater distances the merging of the contributions from all traffic produces a typical urban background value of about 0.5 μg/m³ (Table 7b). In rural areas concentrations are generally less than 0.1 μg/m³.

Table 7a Airborne lead, concentrations near roads

Location	Period	Pb μg/m³ 24h	Daytime only	Notes
M4, central reservation	May–Dec 74	12.3		⎱ 1
Housing area near M4	,,	4.9		⎰
M4 Harlington: 25m from carriageway	11/4/79– 9/7/79	2.2		
95m ,, ,,	,,	0.85		
183m ,, ,,	,,	0.66		
N Circular Rd: 26m ,, ,,	20/4/79–13/7/79	0.93		2
33m ,, ,,	,,	0.55		
71m ,, ,,	,,	0.42		
96m ,, ,,	,,	0.57		
300m ,, ,,	,,	0.42		
Exhibition Rd, SW7	1973		3.2	
Seymour Place, W1	,,		4.0	3
Talgarth Rd, W14	,,		8.8	
Upper Berkeley St, W1	,,		4.3	
Fleet St, EC4, centre	May 62–Feb 63		3.2	4
Fleet St, EC4, centre	Apr 71–Mar 72		6.4	
,,	,, 72– ,, 73	3.3	6.0	5
,,	,, 73– ,, 74	2.8	6.2	
Heath St, Hampstead NW3	,, 72– ,, 73	5.9		
,,	,, 73– ,, 74	5.7		
Clerkenwell Rd, EC1	,, 72– ,, 73		2.8	
,,	,, 73– ,, 74		2.5	
Salford Circus, Birmingham	Jan–Dec 73	1.83		
,,	,, 74	1.46		6
,,	,, 75	1.79		
Perry Barr, outside house by M6	1/3/73–22/3/73	0.98	1.01	
Birmingham, Stratford Rd	Jan–Dec 76	4.1		
,,	,, 77	2.7		
Cardiff, Queen St	Jan–Dec 74	2.5		
,,	,, 75	3.2		
,,	,, 76	1.7		7
Glasgow, Hope St	Jan–Dec 74	2.0		
,,	,, 75	2.5		
,,	,, 76	1.7		
,,	,, 77	2.1		
Warwick, Jury St	Mar 65–Feb 66	3.5		8

Table 7b Airborne lead, concentrations at urban sites

Location	Period	Pb µg/m³ 24h	Daytime only	Notes
St Bartholomew's Med. Coll., EC1	Apr 71–Mar 72		1.5	
,,	,, 72– ,, 73	0.8	1.3	
,,	,, 73– ,, 74	0.7	1.2	5
Chiswick, W4	,, 72– ,, 73	1.3		
,,	,, 73– ,, 74	1.3		
Warwick	Mar 65–Feb 66	0.8		8
Barnsley, town centre	Apr 76–Mar 78	0.36		
Motherwell, town centre	,,	0.46		
Grangemouth, works yard	,,	0.32		
London, Neasden, close to busy road	,,	0.94		
Ellesmere Port, town centre	,,	0.42		
Stoke-on-Trent, behind school	,,	0.31		
Belfast, edge of housing estate	,,	0.31		
Leeds, close to busy road	,,	0.65		
,, city centre	,,	0.51		
,, park	,,	0.27		
Newcastle, old housing area	,,	0.28		9
Coventry, city centre	,,	0.49		
Pembroke Dock, remote area	,,	0.08		
Newport, town centre	,,	0.38		
Bristol, city centre	,,	0.35		
London, busy road, central area	,,	0.72		
Bolton, hospital grounds	,,	0.39		
Sheffield, close to busy road	,,	0.53		
Cambridge, close to busy road	,,	0.48		
Glasgow, close to busy road	,,	0.93		
London – Endell St, WC2	Jan–Dec 73	1.0		
,,	,, 74	0.8		10
,,	,, 75	0.9		
,,	,, 76	0.8		

Table 7c Airborne lead concentrations inside and outside homes

Location	Period	Pb µg/m³ Inside	Outside	%	Notes
Birmingham – house 160m from Salford Circus	29/11/73–19/12/73	0.87	0.88	98	
House alongside M6 at Perry Barr	1/3/74–22/3/74	0.69	0.98	70	6
House with double glazing, M6, Perry Barr	26/4/74–15/5/74	0.44	0.70	63	
First-floor flat,	Apr 72–Mar 73	3.72	5.94	63	5
Heath St, Hampstead	,, 73– ,, 74	3.81	5.70	67	

Table 7—Notes

1 Hogbin and Bevan (1976). The sites were at Harlington, Middlesex (outer London), and the measurements were made in connection with studies on the effects of a noise barrier on the spread of lead emissions. The figures quoted are arithmetic means of a series of 15 observations, with and without barriers in place.

2 Turner and Carroll (1980). The sites were in residential areas adjoining busy roads in outer London, with samplers close to ground level.

3 Harrison *et al* (1974). Spot samples, over period of 30-40 minutes only, were taken as part of a study of the proportion of organic to inorganic lead. The sites were at the kerbside in streets in the inner London area, at a height of 1m.

4 Waller *et al* (1965). Daytime samples were from 08.00–19.00 hours Mondays to Fridays only. The site was an island in the middle of Fleet Street, with the intake at a height of 1.2m.

5 Lawther *et al* (1973), with additional data supplied by the authors. The Fleet Street site was the same as in 4 above. The Clerkenwell Road site was also in central London, about 5m from the road, at a height of 3m. The site at St Bartholomew's Medical College was nearby, about 70m from the road and at a height of 20m. The two other sites were in inner residential areas of London: at Heath Street, Hampstead, outside the window of a first-floor flat, immediately above the pavement at a height of 4m (and with an indoor sampler in the same room) and at Netheravon Road, Chiswick, about 100m from a busy arterial road, at a height of 3m.

6 Department of the Environment (1978). Daytime measurements were from 07.30-19.30 hours. The Salford Circus site was within the large (Gravelly Hill) motorway interchange and the other sites were also adjacent to this junction.

7 Apling *et al* (1979a). The sites were in busy roads in each city, 0.5m from the kerb edge, at a height of 2.5m. In Cardiff and in Glasgow samples were taken on only a limited number of days each year. The street in which the sampler was sited in Cardiff became pedestrianised at the end of 1975.

8 Bullock and Lewis (1968). The street site was in the main thoroughfare (High Street/Jury Street), at a height of 3m, with a further site at the rear of the Council Offices, away from traffic, at a height of 4.5m.

9 McInnes (1979). The sites were chosen to be representative of residential, commercial and industrial areas, at heights between 4 and 25m.

10 Apling *et al* (1979b). This was a laboratory site in a commercial area of central London at a height of 12m. The sampler was moved during 1976 to a similar site by Vauxhall Bridge Road.

Figure 1: Variation of concentrations with distance from motorway

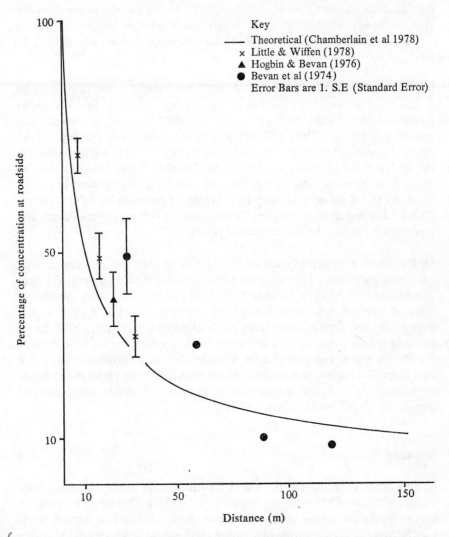

Key
— Theoretical (Chamberlain et al 1978)
× Little & Wiffen (1978)
▲ Hogbin & Bevan (1976)
● Bevan et al (1974)
Error Bars are 1. S.E (Standard Error)

Percentage of concentration at roadside

Distance (m)

59 In view of the large variations in concentration that may occur over short distances, and the extent to which most people move around during the day, it is difficult to estimate true exposures to airborne lead. There may be some exceptional circumstances in which individuals are confined to a locality with relatively high concentrations, but few people are likely to be exposed to long-term average concentrations greater than about 1 $\mu g/m^3$,

29

as indicated by the data in Table 7b. Concentrations of lead in the air inside houses are generally similar to, or a little lower than, those immediately outside. Measurements made in Birmingham, in the vicinity of the Gravelly Hill motorway interchange, and others made in London are shown in Table 7c. These show indoor concentrations ranging from about 60% to 100% of those outside.

60 The total amount of lead emitted to air from traffic varies in proportion to the total consumption of petrol and its lead content. In 1971 about 10,600 tonnes of lead were consumed in petrol and the maximum lead content was 0.84 g/l. Since 1972 it has been UK Government policy to hold the total amount of lead used in petrol constant at the 1971 figure by decreasing the lead content to offset the growth in demand; it has been reduced by stages to its present value of 0.45 g/l, and there is a commitment to reduce it further to 0.4 g/l on 1 January 1981 in accordance with an EEC Directive (Official Journal of the European Communities, 1978) setting maximum and minimum values for the lead content of petrol.

61 Results of a study in Germany in which concentrations of airborne lead have been monitored following the reduction of the lead content of petrol from 0.4 to 0.15 g/l from January 1976 show that, while kerbside concentrations of airborne lead have fallen in proportion with this reduction, the change was less further away from roads (Jost and Sartorius, 1979). There has also been an interesting experiment in Italy where the isotopic ratio of the lead in petrol was changed for a limited period to provide a tracer for lead from that source; the results indicate that lead from petrol is the major contributor to airborne concentrations at urban kerbside sites, but not necessarily elsewhere (Facchetti, 1979).

Industrial Sources

62 Emissions of lead from the major lead industries in the UK have been estimated at 200–250 tonnes per annum (DOE, 1974). This figure is probably an underestimate of the total emission, as lead contained in ferrous scrap may be released on remelting. In addition there are numerous small industries handling and processing lead. Little is known of the emissions of lead to air from these sources. While industrial emissions may not be large on a national scale (representing under 10% of the total emissions) there may be 'hot-spots'. Local problems can arise, for example, from metal recovery operations in small scrap yards, from the burning of old lead-acid battery cases, or from demolition work. Recent measurements of airborne lead near

five of the larger lead works where blood lead concentrations were also determined are given in Table 8. At only one site did the concentration exceed 2 μg/m³; most of the other values were less than 1 μg/m³. In general, at distances greater than 500m, the concentrations had fallen to values similar to or lower than those found in general urban areas.

Table 8 Lead deposition rates and airborne lead concentrations around lead works

Distance (m)		Deposition rates*	Airborne Concentrations
From centre of works	From boundary of works	Pb mg/m² per 30 days 3 month means	Pb μg/m³ 3 month means
Thorpe nr Leeds			
120	40	100	1.2
360	250	17	0.29
990	770	24	0.47
Abbey Wood			
130	25	250	1.8
220	125	210	1.8
465	365	23	0.49
538	445	38	0.59
800	700	14	0.38
Chester			
195	0	140	1.6
315	155	120	2.5
460	275	54	0.72
523	370	46	0.83
985	690	19	0.31
Market Harborough			
215	85	47	0.31
220	90	9	0.14
370	215	18	0.22
390	255	6	0.11
900	750	6	0.14
Gravesend			
465	330	62	1.4
540	505	15	0.70
745	670	13	0.56
820	740	16	0.57

*Measured by standard ISO gauge.
From Turner and Carroll, 1980.

Contribution of Airborne Lead to Deposited Dust

63 Much of the lead in street dust is the result of the fallout of airborne lead but some may also come from weathering of lead paint on houses, street fittings, or yellow lines on the road. This dust must contribute to the amount of lead ingested, particularly by children. Vegetables grown near roads and industrial sources are liable to retain lead deposited on their leaves; in addition the continued fallout year by year of lead from the air onto the ground will increase the concentration of lead in soil and may increase the uptake of lead by plants(see Chapter 2). The importance of each of these possible pathways is not known but they must add somewhat to the effects of inhaled airborne lead. Table 8 gives some figures for deposited lead near lead works. The maximum deposition rates are about 10 times higher than those found near roads, although the airborne concentrations are similar.

64 Table 9 shows the results of measurements of lead in dust in the roadway near the entrance of four lead works. These illustrate the point that the lead content in dust falls off rapidly with increasing distance from the works. Vehicles leaving the premises carry out lead on their tyres, much of which is deposited within a short distance. The significance of these deposits for human exposure is unknown.

Table 9 Lead in dust in the road near lead works

Site	% of lead in dust			
	At Gate	100m	250m	500m
Abbey Wood	7.5	6.8	0.50	0.5–0.9
Chester	2.5–7.2	1.6–6.0	0.25–2.0	0.1–1.7
Market Harborough	3.5–4.0	1.2–2.4	0.1–0.5	0.1
Thorpe (nr Leeds)	7.5	3.5–5	1.2–4	0.25–2.7

From Turner and Carroll, 1980.

5 Adventitious Lead

65 Particular families or individuals may be exposed to sources of lead peculiar to a local environment or a specific product, as distinct from those encountered by the population as a whole in food, water and air. We have termed these sources 'adventitious' and have sought to assess their relative importance and to identify those personal and cultural traits, other than employment in industries dealing with lead and its compounds, which may facilitate such exposure.

66 Most adventitious sources are encountered in or about the home or place of residence and young children are at special risk of exposure. The route of transmission is almost invariably by ingestion either directly, or following the contamination of foodstuffs and beverages. The potential hazards associated with these domestic sources of lead often go unrecognised, particularly by parents and guardians.

67 Exposure derived from adventitious sources may be substantial and markedly in excess of that from lead in the general environment. When such exposures are sustained serious illness and even death may result. In the United Kingdom children are most commonly affected and about 100 cases of childhood lead poisoning are recognised each year.

The Sources of Adventitious Lead

68 The following adventitious sources of lead have been recognised:

a. Paints and primers
b. Dust and soil
c. Glazed and soldered domestic vessels and utensils
d. Eye cosmetics and medicinal preparations from the Indian sub-continent
e. Hair darkening products
f. Metallic lead
g. Miscellaneous

69 Lead compounds have long been used in the manufacture of domestic paints, initially as one of the major ingredients and subsequently as pigments and driers. The amount of lead paint sold has however markedly diminished with advances in paint technology and continues to decline; it has been estimated that leaded paints now make up less than 3% of total sales (involving the use at present rates of some 1500 tonnes of lead each year by UK paintmakers). Most leaded paint is used in the shipbuilding and construction industries. We understand that there is no readily available information on how much leaded paint, if any, is now used in homes or for other consumer purposes, but it is more likely to be applied to exterior surfaces because of its reputation for giving greater protection against weathering. We understand that, as a result of a voluntary agreement between the paint industry and government, paints manufactured in the UK which, for technical reasons, contain more than 1% lead, whether intended for interior or exterior use, are labelled 'Not suitable for use on surfaces liable to be chewed or sucked by children'. In accordance with an adopted EEC Directive (Official Journal of the European Communities, 1977) regulations are to be made requiring appropriate labelling on all paints containing lead in quantities exceeding 0.5% of the total weight. Proprietary lead primers for use on wood are no longer manufactured.

70 Although any hazard from lead in new paint has clearly been substantially reduced, we are concerned that there may still be some risk from lead paint used out-of-doors in places accessible to children or from domestic use of lead paints intended for industry. Warnings on labels are important but are not always effective. We believe that further steps should be taken to complete the elimination of this hazard.

71 In addition, restrictions on the use of lead in new paint cannot eliminate the hazard in all homes since, even when houses are repainted, old paint is seldom completely removed on redecoration and, even if it is, old lead primer may remain in the woodwork beneath. Flakes of paint, which may include old lead-containing layers, may break away or children may chew down to the wood. Old paintwork of high lead content accessible to children continues to be encountered in both public and private housing and in residential institutions and hospitals, although the extent of the problem is unknown. A survey in part of London revealed that over half of the homes visited had accessible paint with a lead content varying between 1% and 40% (Barltrop and Killala, 1969).

72 A small paint flake 2-3mms in diameter may contain over 1000µg of lead or over ten times the daily intake from all other sources (Barltrop and Killala, 1969). The habitual ingestion of such an amount by a child has resulted in severe clinical lead poisoning in 3-4 months (Chisholm and Harrison, 1956). Old lead paintwork in the home is the single most common cause of severe childhood lead poisoning in the United Kingdom and accounts for at least one third of all known cases (Barltrop et al, 1976). McLean (1980) reports that, in England and Wales from 1968 to 1976, 13 children were certified as having died from lead poisoning out of a total of only 46 due to poisoning by all non-medicinal substances other than carbon monoxide; of these 13 deaths 4 were attributed specifically to lead paint.

73 We note that in the United States there is an active programme of lead paint hazard detection and abatement; in 1976, some 500,463 American children were screened for lead poisoning, of whom 69,131 were found to have evidence of undue exposure; 28,333 homes were found to have a lead paint hazard (Billick and Gray, 1978). We believe that steps should be taken in this country to identify housing areas, institutions, schools and play areas where there is a high lead content in existing paintwork. All practicable means should be taken to reduce or eliminate the hazard as soon as possible and research should be be conducted to identify economical and effective methods of doing this.

74 Although the direct ingestion of paint flakes is probably the most important cause of lead poisoning in children, other routes of transmission of lead from paint have been recognised. Degradation of paint film in the home may result in contamination of house dust to which children are also exposed (Vostal et al, 1974); similarly, external paintwork, which may be of greater lead content, may contaminate garden soils immediately adjacent to the home.

75 Painted toys, nursery furniture, pencils, etc, are potential hazards of special importance because of the extent to which they are normally chewed by children. Paints intended for toys are limited by regulation to 0.25% lead and those used on pencils, pens, brushes etc to the stringent limit of 0.025%. Constant vigilance is however essential in the enforcement of these regulations, particularly with regard to imported goods.

Lead in Dust and Soil

76 Many reports implicate lead-contaminated dust and soil as sources of exposure. House dust may be contaminated with lead derived from a variety

of sources in addition to the degradation of paint film; substantial amounts of lead may be liberated in the home at redecoration as a result of sanding, scraping and burning of paint films and may endanger the workers involved as well as the residents of the home (Feldman, 1978). Contaminated industrial clothing improperly brought to the home may carry substantial amounts of lead dust to the domestic environment; the children of some lead smelter workers have been found to have excessive lead burdens which were attributed to this source (Baker *et al*, 1977). However, given full implementation of the existing Codes of Practice for the lead industry, this problem should diminish. Lead may be found in dust as a result of the use of lead-containing cosmetics in the home (paragraphs 79–83) and the burning of lead-containing fuels in fireplaces and heating appliances. The deposition of airborne lead particles from external sources may make a small but detectable contribution.

77 The lead content of soils of gardens and other areas near to the home has received insufficient attention. The blood lead of pre-school children increases by about 0.6 μg/dl for every 1,000 ppm (0.1%) lead in soil (Barltrop, 1975). Enhanced lead levels are encountered particularly in soils in lead mining and lead smelting areas, in land previously used for the deposition of industrial waste and refuse, and in land adjacent to motorways and arterial roads. Concentrations of up to 30,000 ppm of lead in soil have been found in rural villages in old lead mining areas (Barltrop *et al*, 1975). To date there have been no standards for the concentrations of lead to be allowed in soil on land used for housing or similar purposes. The lack of clear guidance has impeded some new housing developments and raised doubts concerning the safety of existing dwellings in some areas. We understand that guidelines are being developed to establish acceptable concentrations of lead in soil in gardens, agricultural land, parks and open spaces. We would support the adoption of such guidelines.

Glazed and Soldered Domestic Utensils

78 Domestic utensils and vessels used for the preparation of foods and beverages may, in certain circumstances, release substantial amounts of lead; regulations have therefore been made prescribing limits for extractable lead from cooking utensils, ceramic and enamelled ware. Imperfections in the glazing of ceramics and earthenware, which can occur with small scale production, may pose a particular hazard. We note that, whereas modern 'pewter' is lead-free, traditional pewter may have a considerable lead content and is still commonly used for drinking beer. The public should be made

aware of the possible hazards of imperfectly glazed ceramic ware and of old pewter. The hazard from lead-contaminated vessels arises particularly where prolonged storage of acid fluids is involved, for example in the fermentation and storage of beers, ciders and wines and in the storage of vinegars, fruits, fruit juices, pickles and preserves.

Eye Cosmetics and Medicines from the Indian Sub-Continent

79 Certain eye cosmetics from the Indian sub-continent contain lead, and members of immigrant communities in particular have been exposed from this source. The cosmetics concerned are the Khols or Surmas, which are applied to the eyes not only of adults, but also of children and infants. In earlier times they were formulated from antimony sulphide but in recent years economic factors have resulted in the use of lead in some preparations. Surmas are described as being white, grey or black. Our information is that the grey and black forms are likely to contain a large proportion of lead. The Pharmacy Department of the University of Nottingham report that Surmas may include up to 83% lead (Table 10).

Table 10 Chemical analysis of proprietary Surmas sold or brought into the United Kingdom but manufactured in India or Pakistan

Description	Powder colour	Percentage lead
Hashmi Surma Jowahar Chaharam, Karachi	Grey	80.2
Surma Moqawi Basar Taj Company, Lahore	Grey	53.7
Multani, Ayurvedic 36-H Connaught Circus, Delhi	Grey	Trace
Nag Jyoti, Murrari Brothers, Delhi	White	Trace (Zinc 4.5% + Menthol)
MD Hashim Surma, Bunder Road, Karachi	Grey	82.9
Bal Jyoti, Murrari Brothers, Delhi	Grey-Black	38.4
Indian Surma	Cream	Trace
Bhimsaini Kajal with Aela, Murrari Brothers, Delhi	Black Paste	Trace
Nargasi Surma, Hamdard, Pakistan	Grey	77.3
Binger Surma, Hamdard, Pakistan	Black	26.3
*Bhimsaini Kajal with Aela	Black Paste	Trace

Trace = <0.5%
*Carbon in soft paraffin base.
From Aslam *et al* (1979)

80 In 1968 the Home Office sought a voluntary ban on the sale of lead-containing cosmetics. We are pleased to learn that more recently the Cosmetic

Products Regulations 1978, which implement an EEC Directive, have made the sale of lead-containing cosmetics in the course of business illegal. The use of lead acetate in hair care products is the only permitted exception. It appears that private imports of lead-containing cosmetics continue however and that use of these cosmetics is still a practice among immigrant families from the Indian sub-continent.

81 It is inevitable that there will be some absorption of lead from preparations such as Surma, particularly due to children sucking contaminated fingers. It seems that the use of Surma may be widespread and we are concerned that children may be seriously exposed in this way.

82 There are some reports of acute lead poisoning which have been attributed to Surma; it seems, however, that in homes where Surma is used there are commonly other sources of lead which may have played a part in the poisoning (Fernandes, 1969; Warley *et al*, 1968). Although studies of immigrant children (Josephs, 1977; Ali *et al*, 1978) indicate that the blood lead levels of those children who use Surma are significantly higher than of those who do not, we consider that Surma has not been proved to be the only cause of this difference. Studies by Waldron (1979a) and unpublished work by Ali *et al* and Archer *et al* indicate that in this country blood lead concentrations of women and children are significantly higher in those of Asian extraction than in others.

83 We consider that the private importation and use of lead-containing cosmetics is unsafe and should be strongly discouraged. Potential users of these products should be made aware of the hazard.

84 Some unlicensed medicinal products prescribed by practitioners of traditional Indian medicine (the Hakims or Vaids) contain lead. Poisoning has been reported from the use of purported aphrodisiacs containing lead (Brearley and Forsythe, 1978). Formulations of several medicines which contain large amounts of lead and other metals are given in Table 11. The nature and use of these medicines are being investigated. Action to educate those concerned about the hazards of traditional remedies containing lead is, we understand, already in hand.

Hair Darkening Products

85 Some hair darkening products on the market have contained lead acetate in concentrations ranging from 0.26–3.13%. Waldron (1979b) reports that

Table 11 Heavy metal impurities in some medicines from the Indian sub-Continent

	Impurities		
	Major Component	Minor Component	Trace Component
Khamira gaozaban			Zn 130 ppm contained with 41% dextrose and silver particles
Female fertility stimulant, silver coated			Silver
Male fertility stimulant, orange brown, pliable mass			Zn 168 ppm contained in 15% sucrose together with vegetable matter
Maha sudarshan. Churna powder		Iron	Titanium, manganese, zinc, rubidium, strontium
Cogoni oil			Iron, zinc
Bajar, used by men and women	(Nicotine)		Manganese, iron, zinc, lead, copper
Queen's balm			Zinc
Bala guti pills (useful for children's diseases)			Lead 58 ppm, antimony 750 ppm, arsenic 2 ppm
Hari taki tablets			Iron, zinc, rubidium
Chandraprapha pills	Iron	Titanium, chromium, manganese, nickel, zinc, arsenic, strontium	
Terminalia chebula powder	Zinc, rubidium	Iron	
Pushyanug churna powder		Iron	Titanium, manganese, nickel, zinc, arsenic, strontium, lead
Khadiradi pills		Iron	Titanium, manganese, copper, zinc, rubidium, strontium
Withania somnifera		Iron	Titanium, manganese, zinc, arsenic (2 ppm), strontium
Marayan churna			Manganese, zinc, strontium

After Aslam *et al*, (1979).

ingestion of a quantity of one of these preparations was responsible for a case of lead poisoning in a young West Indian girl in Birmingham. The Cosmetic Products Regulations 1978 restrict the use of lead acetate in hair darkening products to a maximum concentration of 3% and require the following instructions to be given to users: 'Wash hands after use. Do not use on broken or abraded skin. Keep out of reach of children'. There is no compulsion on the manufacturers to state that their product contains lead, although a few of them do so. In our opinion all hair darkening products which contain lead should have this stated clearly on the label of the container, together with the warning against their misuse.

Metallic Lead and Miscellaneous Sources

86 The use of car battery casings as fuel in domestic fires and heaters is an occasional cause of lead poisoning (Chisholm and Barltrop, 1979). Fuel 'logs' made from coloured newsprint have been reported to release lead when burnt. Children who habitually chew coloured newsprint to produce 'spitballs' have been found to have raised lead levels. Certain hobbies, including the making of jewellery or stained glass, may be dangerous. Metallic lead is not normally hazardous and to swallow a single lead-containing item is unlikely to be harmful unless it is sufficiently large to be retained in the stomach. The ingestion by children of many small pieces of lead such as lead shot, fishing weights or curtain weights, has caused lead poisoning.

Pica

87 Pica is defined as the ingestion of substances not normally regarded as foodstuffs. Its potential as a contributory cause of lead poisoning is very clear. Pica has been recognised among adults for centuries, notably as an occasional feature of pregnancy but also as a manifestation of extreme hunger. The term pica is an allusion to the magpie (Pica pica pica (linn)), which is said to have an appetite which is both capricious and voracious. A variant of pica known as geophagia (earth-eating) was described by Livingstone and by Van Hambold and Bonfland in the natives of Africa and South America respectively. These and other historical reports have been reviewed in a classical monograph by Cooper (1957).

88 The occurrence of pica in childhood has been recognised only during the last few decades. Cooper (1957) surveyed 784 children and noted that pica was present in 21.9% and that it was rare after the age of six years. It has been suggested that pica is more common in negro than in white children (Cooper, 1957; Dickins and Ford, 1942; Millican et al, 1962) but Barltrop (1966) found no significant difference in the prevalence of pica in white

compared with negro children in a randomly selected population, stratified for ethnic group. Many attempts have been made to determine the aetiology of pica in childhood. Thus Lanzkowsky (1959) related pica to concomitant iron deficiency and other authors have implicated several other mineral deficiency states. However, Gutelius *et al* (1962) and Gutelius (1963), in controlled supplementation trials, failed to confirm the role of nutritional deficiencies. Millican *et al* (1956) attributed the practice to a disturbed mother-child relationship and Lourie *et al* (1958) suggested that it represented an early pattern of addiction. Barltrop (1966) noted that the practice was commonplace and inversely related to age in the range one to six years and he therefore suggested that pica was a normal manifestation of development. Recently, Bicknell (1975) reported studies on children in hospital and found pica to be related to a low mental age, the presence of additional handicaps and behavioural disturbances. She argued that selective and highly motivated pica represented a maladaptive behaviour pattern rather than a developmental phenomenon.

Pica and Lead Paint

89 Numerous reports of pica involving lead based paint have appeared in the literature and it is still regarded as a most important aetiological factor for severe clinical lead poisoning in childhood. It is standard procedure to record the presence or absence of pica in paediatric practice and to X-ray the abdomen for evidence of ingested paint flakes in suspected cases of lead poisoning. Several authors have advocated that enquiries should be made for pica as a means for the detection of childhood lead poisoning. A positive history of pica in 94% of 30 cases of clinical lead poisoning in childhood has been reported by Tanis (1955). Similarly, Bradley *et al* (1956) in a study of 604 children found that 69.6% of those with blood lead concentrations of $50\mu g/dl$ or more gave a history of pica. On the other hand, Greenberg *et al* (1958) found evidence of lead poisoning in only 24% of 194 children with pica. Griggs *et al* (1964) argued that knowledge of the place of residence is a more helpful diagnostic aid than a history of pica. More sensitive and more specific methods for screening populations of children for lead poisoning have now been developed although they have yet to be applied generally in the United Kingdom.

6 Uptake of Lead

90 Earlier chapters have reviewed what is known of the amounts of lead which people may ingest from food and water, the concentrations of lead in air to which they may be exposed and the additional sources which may contribute to the exposure of some individuals. In this chapter we shall consider the extent to which lead is absorbed by different routes and retained by the body, in order to assess the relative importance of the different sources of lead.

The Absorption and Fate of Lead in the Body

91 Lead enters the body primarily by absorption from the gastrointestinal tract of a proportion of ingested lead and by absorption from the lower respiratory tract of the proportion of inhaled airborne lead which is retained there. Further details of these routes are given in paragraphs 96–108. A proportion of airborne lead which is trapped in the upper respiratory tract is removed to the throat by ciliary action and may be swallowed. Having gained access to the blood, the lead is carried on the surface of the red cells, quickly reaching higher concentrations in whole blood than in serum or extracellular fluid generally. Lead is stored in and mobilised from bone and teeth in a similar way to calcium. Some lead is stored in soft tissues but in adults some 95% of the total amount of lead in the body is in bone, the proportion being somewhat lower in children. The amount of lead in bone tends to increase through adult life, whereas the amount in soft tissues tends to remain constant. Lead is excreted in both urine and faeces, that in the latter being due to unabsorbed lead as well as to lead positively excreted from the biliary tract; under some circumstances the total amount of lead excreted exceeds the total of that ingested plus that absorbed from the respiratory tract. Blood lead tends to reach equilibrium within about 2-3 months of a change in exposure but it is uncertain whether equilibrium between bone and blood is ever reached; blood lead therefore tends to reflect recent rather than long term exposure. The relationship between the concentrations of

lead in blood and in soft tissues after critical exposure is not known, although they are presumed to move together. Lead crosses the placentral barrier freely and concentrations tend to be similar in mothers and in their new born babies.

92 The effects of lead may be thought of as a continuous spectrum having normality at one extreme, passing through absorption of lead with no detectable change, to absorption with detectable biochemical change of uncertain significance for health and, finally, to poisoning with the presence of symptoms and signs at the other extreme (Windeyer Report, 1972).

93 The contribution of a given source to lead in the body is usually expressed as the concentration of lead in the blood due to that source. Ideally, one would use the amount of lead in the entire body, or the concentration of lead in the parts of the body of most concern (such as the brain) instead of blood lead but this information can obviously be obtained only by post mortem examination; difficulties would in any case arise with the use of any measure of the total body burden of lead, since it represents the net accumulation of lead over a lifetime and information on the exposures which had contributed to it would never be available in practice. In studies of the clinical effects of past exposure to lead, on the other hand, measures of the total body burden are useful; tooth lead concentrations are believed to give a reasonably accurate reflection of long term exposure and, since children can be persuaded to give their deciduous teeth for research, tooth lead is becoming widely used in studies of this type. Hair accumulates lead and should in theory represent exposure in the medium term but the techniques which are available for analysing lead in hair are not yet sufficiently developed; there are major problems with these techniques, especially in the standardisation of sampling procedures and in separating lead which has contaminated the hair surface from that stored within the hair. Blood lead is widely regarded as the best available indicator of recent exposure to lead and it is thus appropriate for use in studies of the relative importance of the lead to which people are currently exposed from different parts of the environment.

94 Three types of study are available in the literature which help to determine these relative contributions. First are experiments in which individuals are exposed to varying but known amounts of lead through the air they breathe or by ingestion, and their blood lead concentrations are determined. Such studies commonly involve very high exposures of uncertain relevance to everyday life and can be conducted only on small numbers of volunteers; the results may therefore be dominated by individual variations in response. Second are 'balance studies' in which the lead excreted in faeces and urine,

as well as the lead ingested, is assessed and the net gain or loss of lead calculated. Studies can combine features of both these first two types. A variant involves labelling experimentally administered lead with a radioactive isotope, which allows the distribution of the dosed lead within the body to be studied. Third are epidemiological surveys in which concentrations of lead occurring in the environment are studied and linked with observations on blood lead amongst samples of the population. Such studies have generally been conducted on populations thought to be specially at risk (the so-called 'target' populations), particularly from high levels of lead in water, and they have not taken account of lead in more than one part of the environment. The results of studies of these kinds which have been undertaken in relation to ingested and inhaled lead, in adults and in children, are reviewed in paragraphs 96 to 108.

95 No studies have been undertaken which provide direct and accurate data on lead in all parts of the environment to which a study population has been exposed. We have therefore examined data on blood lead drawn from samples of the general population in particular areas in relation to estimates of representative levels of lead for the same localities. Appropriate blood lead data have become available recently from survey work in the United Kingdom to implement the EEC Directive on Biological Screening of the Population for Lead (paragraph 110, Table 12 and Appendix 2).

Experiments and Balance Studies: Lead by Ingestion

96 Kehoe (1961, a, b, c, and d), Rabinowitz *et al* (1974) and Hursh and Suomela (1968) have carried out isotope studies involving the ingestion of ^{203}Pb or ^{212}Pb by adult volunteers. The studies indicated an average absorption rate of 11% although the number of individuals studied was small. Both Blake (1976) and Barltrop and Strehlow (1978) undertook balance studies and found a very wide range of absorption rates amongst adults, with some individuals being in overall negative balance. It has been generally accepted that the average net absorption of ingested lead by adults is 10%. The absorption factor is not constant, even for an individual, but depends upon such factors as amounts of fat, minerals (particularly calcium) and vitamins (Barltrop and Khoo, 1976) in the diet and the physical and chemical form of the lead. Experiments show that absorption of lead is somewhat greater when lead is ingested (eg in water) between rather than with meals but there is no direct evidence on the absorption of lead from tap water in normal circumstances. It is reasonable to assume for present purposes that all ingested lead is absorbed to a similar extent whatever the source.

97 There are three groups of experimental or related theoretical studies which deal with the relationship of ingested lead and blood lead. In theoretical studies based on the absorption factor discussed above, Chamberlain *et al* (1978) predicted that the increase in blood lead concentration per 100 µg/day of lead in the diet would be 3.6 µg/dl; assumptions were also made concerning the fraction of uptake from the gut that is transferred to red cells and the biological half-life of lead in blood. The results from four experimental studies cited by Chamberlain (involving only 17 subjects in all) show an average increase in blood lead concentrations per 100 µg/day of lead intake of 1.99 µg/dl and a range of 1.4–4.3 µg/dl. In studies of three subjects using [204]Pb as a tracer, the proportions of blood lead attributed to current diet were 53, 53, and 75% respectively (Rabinowitz *et al*, 1976). The remainder of the blood lead was reported as being due not only to intake from other sources, mainly by inhalation, but also to resorption from storage in bone.

98 Ethical considerations limit work on children to the use of balance studies. Eleven such studies were carried out by Alexander *et al* (1973) on eight normal children aged 3 months to 8½ years. They showed an average intake of 10.61 µg/kg/day and an average absorption (ie intake less faecal excretion) of 5.47 µg/kg/day (52%); there was wide variation between individuals. Recently Ziegler *et al* (1978) carried out a number of three day balance studies on each of nine infants aged 2 weeks to 2 years, who were on ordinary diets. Average intake was 10.29 µg/kg/day and average absorption was 4.39 µg/kg/day (43%). In a second series of studies Ziegler *et al* (1978) showed that the proportion of intake which is absorbed is very dependent on the dose; infants on diets providing low intakes of less than 5 µg/kg/day were in negative balance.

99 In longer-term balance studies in 29 hospitalised children, who may not necessarily reflect the response of children living in their normal environment, Barltrop and Strehlow (1978) found that a considerable number of children given hospital diets, duplicate samples of which were analysed for lead, were in negative balance. Wide individual variations in net retention of lead were observed ranging from a negative balance of 57% to a positive balance of 99%, with an average negative balance of approximately 40% of the dietary intake in children ranging in age from 3 weeks to 14 years.

100 To allow the uptake of lead by children from food and water to be compared with that from air, assumptions must be made about average intake and average proportion absorbed. Because the proportion of lead absorbed varies so greatly, estimates of the average absorption based on studies of small numbers of children must be treated with caution, but it is clear that

the proportion absorbed is much greater in children than in adults; in our calculations we shall assume 40% absorption. Paragraph 17 quotes an estimate of lead intake based on national dietary studies in 2–4 year old children. The figure of 70–80 µg/day is roughly equivalent to 5.5 µg/kg/day, which is substantially less than reported from the balance studies. We shall assume an intake of 8 µg/kg/day and hence an absorption of 3.2 µg/kg/day, when making a comparison with inhaled lead in paragraph 114.

Epidemiological Surveys:

101 Surveys of lead in water and blood lead were reviewed by Berlin *et al* (1977). Leaving aside the results of Moore *et al* (1977a) which are discussed below, the range of results was 0.7–3.4 µg/dl blood lead per 100 µg/l water lead, with a median of 1.3 and an unweighted mean of 1.8. Assuming an average intake of 1.25 l/day (Table 5 and paragraph 49) this corresponds to a range of 0.5–2.8 µg/dl blood lead per 100 µg/day ingested water lead with a median of 1.1 and a mean of 1.5. These figures are lower than those reported from experimental and theoretical work quoted in paragraph 97 but the difference may be largely explained by the use of first draw water samples in many of the surveys.

102 Individual studies have not been large enough for the form of the relation between water lead and blood lead to be examined. However, Moore *et al* (1977a) collated data from a number of Scottish studies and reported that mean blood lead concentrations tend to rise in a curvilinear manner as illustrated by Line A of Figure 2. A damping of the effect on blood lead as water lead rises can be seen. The actual regression equation derived from the data expressed in µmols/1 is as follows:

Mean blood lead $= 0.533 + 0.675^3 \sqrt{\text{first draw water lead}}$

103 Thomas *et al* (1979) derived a similar curve, illustrated by Line B of Figure 2, from their study of a small community in North Wales mentioned in paragraph 43. Two adjacent housing estates, one with lead plumbing and one with copper plumbing, both received the same highly plumbosolvent water. Water leads in the lead-plumbed estate were exceptionally high, with a median concentration of 1,075 µg/l and a maximum of 2,826 µg/l in first draw samples. The median blood lead concentrations among people living in the lead-plumbed houses, at about 38 µg/dl, were more than twice those of people in the houses with copper plumbing; the maximum individual figure recorded was 68 µg/dl. A special feature of this study was that the opportunity

46

arose to study the effect on blood lead of a substantial reduction in environmental lead when all the lead pipes were replaced; the mean blood lead concentrations then declined in the previously lead-plumbed estate by about 50% within six months, confirming that very high water lead has a marked effect on blood lead.

104 Caution is needed in defining the precise form of the relationship derived in these studies. That of Thomas *et al* (1979) was based on relatively few people; Moore *et al* (1977a) themselves point out that their data were drawn from a number of studies and do not represent any one defined population. It seems likely that the extent of the increase in blood lead which results from small increases of water lead, especially from a low initial level, will depend on the size of the intake from other sources such as food. Nevertheless it is safe to conclude from these studies that the relationship between ingested lead and blood lead is curvilinear.

The Effect of Ingested Lead on Blood Lead

105 Estimates of the factor linking blood lead to ingested lead vary considerably. The increases in blood lead per 100 μg/day of ingested lead, estimated from experiments, range from 1.4 to 4.3 μg/dl blood lead (paragraph 97); estimates from surveys are reasonably compatible. From the results and from theoretical work, Chamberlain *et al* (1978) suggested a factor of 3.5 μg/dl blood lead per 100 μg/day ingested lead. All these estimates however are based on the assumption of a linear relationship and we have seen (paragraphs 102 to 104) that this is unlikely to be correct. The implications of a curvilinear relationship can be demonstrated by making some calculations from the regression equation of Moore *et al* (1977a) although, for reasons set out in paragraph 104, it would be unjustified to rely on the exact figures obtained. It can be calculated using the equation that a small increase of lead by ingestion increases blood lead at the rate of approximately 7 μg/dl of blood lead per 100 μg/day ingested lead when starting from a baseline of 18 μg/dl blood lead; of approximately 2 μg/dl blood lead per 100 μg/day ingested lead from a baseline of 24 μg/dl blood lead; and of approximately 1 μg/dl blood lead per 100 μg/day ingested lead from a baseline of 30 μg/dl blood lead. It thus seems likely that the factor linking blood lead to ingested lead is higher at common levels of lead in the environment than has been calculated from experimental work and from surveys on highly exposed populations. The existence of a curvilinear relationship may well explain why factors derived from research work do not fully account for blood lead concentrations as found in the general population (Chamberlain

et al, 1978) and may help to explain the great range of factors reported from different studies. At the same time, it makes the assessment of the relative importance of different sources of lead difficult; this question is taken up again in paragraphs 109–113.

Inhaled Lead

106 The determination of the contribution that airborne lead makes to the total uptake of lead is complex, since it depends not only on the volume of air breathed and the average concentration of lead to which a person is exposed, but also on the extent to which the particles are retained in the respiratory tract and on how much of the lead is then absorbed into the blood. Retention and absorption are markedly affected by the physical and chemical characteristics of the particles, and since many of these present in the air are complex aggregates (as noted in paragraph 56) they are liable to behave differently from the regularly shaped particles on which classical laboratory experiments on the retention of lead have been based. Studies which deal specifically with particulate lead as it actually occurs in the atmosphere and which include measurements of blood lead are therefore required to investigate the contribution of airborne lead.

107 The results of extensive investigations on the retention and absorption of lead as present in the particulate emissions from a small petrol engine have been reported by Chamberlain *et al* (1978). The lead alkyl in the petrol was labelled with a radioactive isotope so that the exhaust products could be traced when inhaled by volunteer subjects. From their observations the authors were able to calculate a factor which they referred to as α, representing the increment in blood lead (in μg/dl) corresponding with each μg/m³ of lead in the air that they breathed. This is analogous with the factor which relates blood and ingested lead, discussed in paragraph 105. The mean value of α that they reported was about 2, but there was a wide scatter in results among the small number of volunteers studied. There is no reason to suppose that the value of α will be constant over the whole range of air lead concentrations to which man is exposed and every reason to assume from experience of occupational exposures to high concentrations that it is not (Richter *et al*, 1979). All the evidence indicates that the value of α falls as the concentration in air rises (Hammond *et al*, 1979), although the form of the equation relating blood lead to air lead has not been defined clearly. Similar findings for ingested lead are reported in paragraphs 102 and 103. Some support for a value of α around 2 within the range of air lead concentrations found in urban atmospheres comes however from the work of Azar *et al*

48

(1975) in which personal samplers were used to assess exposures from the general air, and from that of Griffin *et al* (1975) in which adults were exposed to artificially produced lead aerosols in an experimental chamber. In view of the diversity of concentrations and forms of lead aerosols involved in all these studies, doubts must remain about the most appropriate value of α for the circumstances prevailing in the general air, but for the purpose of assessing the effects of airborne lead in the concentrations normally found in British cities it may be accepted as 2; an annual mean concentration of airborne lead of 1 μg/m^3 then represents a contribution of 2 μg/dl to the concentration of lead in blood. \

108 Ethical constraints prevent experimental studies and epidemiological work involving the taking of blood from children, unless it is thought that they may be at risk. In the case of children not exposed to abnormal levels of lead, calculations can be made based on studies employing a variety of physiological measurements and assumptions, although these studies lack the direct and detailed experimental verification that is possible in adults. Using the calorie requirements for young children which were set out in Table 1, it may be calculated that the ventilation rate during the first three years of life is 0.49m^3/kg body weight/day. No measurements have been reported on the proportional deposition of lead aerosols in the lungs of children. The airways in young children are smaller and their respiratory rate is greater than in adults. James (1977) has calculated that in a ten year old child the percentage retention of very small particles will be slightly higher than in adults so that it is reasonable to assume that 70% of an inhaled lead aerosol is deposited in the lower respiratory tract of children and that, as with adults, 100% of deposited lead will be absorbed. From all this information, it can be assumed that the equivalent volume of air from which lead is taken up per day by the young child is 0.34m^3/kg body weight.

The Relative Contribution of the Different Sources to Blood Lead

109 The relative contributions of the different sources of lead in the environment will be estimated from recent data on blood lead and from the information on amounts of lead in the environment which was given in earlier chapters. A number of uncertainly based assumptions have to be made and the results can indicate only the approximate relative importance of each source for that part of the urban population which face no special exposures; the effect of 'hot-spots' will not be reflected in these estimates.

110 Data on the blood lead concentrations of adults in six English cities have been taken from the results of surveys carried out in the UK in 1979 as part of the EEC programme of blood lead surveillance and they are shown in Table 12. In these surveys samples of adults had been selected in accordance with good statistical practice as being representative of those who live in the cities in question but who are not known to have any abnormal exposure to lead. Analysis of the blood samples was strictly monitored by an international quality control scheme. (Details of the programme and the results of the surveys carried out in the UK are given in Appendix 2.)

Table 12   Blood lead concentrations in 6 cities

	Geometric Mean, μg/dl		
	Inner City	Outer City	Differences
London	12.0[1]	10.2[1,2]	1.8
Birmingham	13.6	11.1	1.5
Leeds	15.6	13.3	2.3
Sheffield	14.6	13.2	1.4
Liverpool	14.2	13.8[2]	0.4
Manchester	17.0	16.6	0.4
6 cities	12.8[1]	11.0[1,2]	1.8

[1] Weighted by total number of electors in each area surveyed.
[2] Adjusted for sex bias.

111 Table 12 shows that the blood lead concentrations of inner city adults are higher on average than those of outer city adults; the differences vary from 0.4–2.3 μg/dl and representative values for the mean blood lead concentrations of inner and outer city adults are assessed as 12.8 and 11.0 μg/dl respectively. These means are heavily weighted towards the London figures because of the size of London's population. The differences in mean blood lead concentrations between cities may be partly accounted for by differences in water lead; none of the cities is recognised as having a major problem with plumbosolvent water but London has virtually no lead in tap water whereas Manchester has somewhat raised levels and the other cities for which there is some information have intermediate levels. (DoE, unpublished.)

112 We have assumed that the estimates of the range of the national average adult intake from food of 70 to 150 μg/day reported in paragraph 24 can be applied to these cities. Water lead is very unevenly distributed but from such

Table 13 Estimated contributions of sources of lead to body burden of adults

		Inner City		Suburbs	
Lead in environment	Water	0 & 50 μg/l	a	0 & 50 μg/l	a
	Air	1.0 μg/m³	b	0.5 μg/m³	c
Intake of lead per day	Food	70 & 150 μg	d	70 & 150 μg	d
	Water	0 & 62.5 μg	e	0 & 62.5 μg	e
Mean blood lead		12.8 μg/dl	f	11.0 μg/dl	f
Blood lead from air		2.0 μg/dl (16%)	g	1.0 μg/dl (9%)	g
Blood lead from food	Water lead=0	84%	h	91%	h
	Food lead =70 μg/d Water lead=50 μg/l	44%	i	48%	i
	Food lead =150 μg/d Water lead= 50 μg/l	59%	i	64%	i
Blood lead from water	Water lead=0	0		0	
	Food lead =70 μg/d Water lead=50 μg/l	40%	i	43%	i
	Food lead =150 μg/d Water lead= 50 μg/l	25%	i	27%	i

NOTES

a From paras 51 & 112.

b From paras 59 & 112.

c From paras 58 & 112.

d From paras 24 & 112.

e Assuming mean consumption 1.25 l/day of water (including contribution from cooking) From (a), para 49 and Table 5.

f From para 111 and Table 12.

g Assuming $\alpha=2$ – From (b), (c), (f) and para 107.

h 100% less percentage at (g).

i Assumes Water Lead and Food Lead are absorbed similarly. Calculated as follows and similarly:

eg $\dfrac{70}{70+62.5} \times 84\% = 44\%$

information as is available we have assessed the range of concentrations in these cities to be approximately 0–50 $\mu g/1$; the great majority of the inhabitants will be exposed to little lead in water. We have taken the 'typical urban background value' for air lead of 0.5 $\mu g/m^3$ reported in paragraph 58 as applying as an average to suburban areas; so as to avoid any risk of underestimating the importance of air lead in inner city areas, we have used as an average for those areas the figure of 1 $\mu g/m^3$, although it should be noted that this figure is quoted in paragraph 59 as a concentration to which few people are likely to be exposed as a long term average.

113 The assumption that the relationship between ingested lead and blood lead is linear has been shown to be incorrect but we do not have adequate data from which to support the use of a curvilinear relationship. In the face of this difficulty we have proceeded by apportioning the mean blood lead concentrations for the six cities between the main sources, on the following basis. The proportion of the observed blood lead which is due to air lead was first calculated on the basis of the estimated concentrations of 0.5 and 1.0 $\mu g/m^3$, and a value of 2 for α. The remainder was then apportioned between food and water, assuming in turn the maximum and minimum concentrations set out in paragraph 112. Calculations are set out in Table 13. They suggest in round terms that adults living in cities who are not specially exposed to lead derive from 45–90% of their blood lead from food, 0–45% from water and 10-20% from air.

114 Data on blood lead in concentrations in representative samples of children who are not specially exposed to lead are not available, so that calculations have to depend upon estimates of absorption rates. Using the figures for absorption of ingested and inhaled lead quoted in paragraphs 100 and 108, the estimate of dietary intake also given in paragraph 100 and the assumptions about lead in air and water given in paragraph 112, our calculations suggest in round terms that children living in cities who are not specially exposed to lead derive 55–95% of their blood lead from food, 0–40% from water and 3–10% from air. The lower proportion from air compared with adults depends upon the assumption that rates of absorption from the intestine are very much higher in children than in adults.

115 The above results assume no mineralisation of garden soil and no intake from paint, dust or other adventitious sources. Such assumptions may not be correct, particularly for dwellers in inner cities. The mean difference in blood lead concentrations between dwellers in inner and outer city areas as indicated by the EEC Surveys is 1.8 $\mu g/dl$ which is slightly more than would be predicted from the likely differences in air lead. These city

dwellers are not subject to major industrial emissions of lead but an additional source may be lead paint, which is regularly found in the older housing stock of these areas. If lead paint does affect adults it must be by the dust derived from it blowing onto food which is insufficiently cleansed before it is eaten. Some effect of this kind cannot be excluded but it does not seem likely that it is a significant source of pollution to adults except in special and localised circumstances. The difference in blood lead concentrations between dwellers in inner and outer city areas is as great in London as elsewhere which suggests that differences in water lead cannot account for it.

Some Special Exposures

116 Sources of exceptionally high exposure for children have been reviewed in earlier chapters and especially in Chapter 5 (Adventitious Sources). Much has been published on the body burden of individual children with overt poisoning but there are relatively few data on the burden of lead of populations of children who may be at special risk. Some findings which have been published are reviewed below.

117 Many surveys of children living close to leadworks in the United Kingdom have been undertaken during the past decade. Recently 16 surveys have been carried out under the EEC programme on children living close to lead industries or in a leadworkers' family; the details are in Appendix 2. Most of the groups of children studied readily met the EEC criteria for blood lead in populations but three groups did not. Local factors which enhance exposure to lead have been identified in these cases and appropriate action is being taken. There was a difference of 2.9 µg/dl in mean blood lead concentrations between a sub group living close to a leadworks and another living further away in one survey, and a difference of 3.0 µg/dl in another. From earlier work the effect of distance is still noticeable at 0.5 km but has disappeared by 1 km.

118 Some of the EEC surveys dealt specifically with leadworkers' children. The effect of living in a leadworker's house varies. In one survey the mean blood lead of such children was 17.4 µg/dl, compared with 16 and 12.1 µg/dl for two groups of neighbouring children. In another, the difference was only 1 µg/dl for boys and 1.5 µg/dl for girls. We know of no explanation of the increased blood lead in these children other than a build up of lead in the home environment due to lead taken home by the worker on his person or his car.

119 Other surveys carried out under the EEC programme dealt with both adults and children living near to busy road junctions and motorways. The results show that blood lead concentrations are within the recommended reference levels, though there are indications that in some localities contributions from traffic increases blood lead concentrations.

120 There is evidence that children living in areas where the soil is contaminated with lead experience an increase in their mean blood lead concentration that is proportional to the amount of lead in the soil. Barltrop *et al* (1975) estimate that blood lead increases by 0.6 µg/dl for each 1,000 ppm of lead in soil. Factors that influence this increase, other than soil lead levels, have not been identified. Barltrop (1975) did not find a similar correlation for adults.

121 Lead in drinking water may have a marked effect on body burden in the case of artificially fed infants in areas where the water lead is exceptionally high (Table 6). A study is in progress in Glasgow, where some households have markedly raised levels of lead in tapwater, to assess this problem and the first results that are available to us suggest that in many cases the infants are ingesting an undesirably large amount of lead. There are as yet insufficient data to confirm this or to allow the implications to be assessed. The field work for this study is due to be completed by April 1980.

122 In the United States old lead paint in poorly maintained property has long been recognised as a major source of lead for young children. A large scale screening programme has been in progress for many years, in which blood lead measurements have been made on over one and a half million children, to identify those at risk and to take remedial action where necessary. In a recent report (Billick and Gray, 1978), the accumulated results were considered in relation to ethnic origins and other factors and it was noted that the overall trends in seasonal mean blood lead values for New York showed some similarity to those in air lead concentrations over the same period. When the same blood lead data were considered in relation to trends in the amount of lead in gasoline sold in the region there was an even closer correlation (Billick *et al*, 1979). This does not necessarily imply a causal relationship and it would be surprising if it did, for at the individual level it is clear that paint is responsible for the more extreme blood lead values. One possible explanation is that since this is specifically a long term screening exercise rather than a survey of random populations there could well be a tendency for the worst cases to be sought first, producing a decline in the mean value over the years, and the peaks seen in summer could reflect a greater exposure of children to dusts then, or special efforts in the more

favourable weather to seek out those at risk. The downward trend in lead from gasoline observed is probably related to the increased use of lead free grades in the New York area and the increased amount in summer may reflect greater consumption during holiday periods. These points may become clearer when further details of the study are published.

123 A very careful study of the distribution of blood lead concentrations among school children in Sydney, New South Wales, has been reported recently (Garnys et al, 1979). Mean values were higher among children at two schools in an urban area than among those in a rural area and, while it was possible to attribute some extreme values to the ingestion of flaking paint, the authors considered that the overall differences between the groups were related to airborne lead. One surprising feature of the results was that many values in the urban group were higher than those reported in most of the recent EEC surveys in the United Kingdom, despite the apparently more limited opportunities for intake of lead from tap water and old paint. From the information available, concentrations of airborne lead did not appear to be higher in Sydney than they are in similar places in the United Kingdom. The assessment of exposure in this study was not detailed enough to allow any quantitative relationship between blood lead and airborne lead to be calculated and the relatively high blood lead values must be regarded as unexplained.

Conclusions

124 The main purpose of this chapter of the report has been to assess the importance of the different sources of lead to which the population of the United Kingdom as a whole are exposed. The importance to the population of the main environmental sources is, in descending order, food, water and air; although our calculations are based in part on uncertain assumptions, this general conclusion is clear. Special consideration has been given to the importance of lead derived from vehicle emissions and we estimate that in city dwellers it may account for between 10 and 20% of blood lead. The contribution of dust and other adventitious sources to the exposure of the population as a whole is not known but we have found no reason to conclude that it is a major factor.

125 No firm evidence exists for guidance on what might be taken as a wholly 'safe' level in the environment or the body. After considering the available data, the Commission of the European Communities has suggested 'reference levels' for blood lead in members of the general population. Under the terms

of the recent Directive (CEC, 1977) surveys of blood lead levels are required to determine the distribution of values in samples of the population in each member country; remedial action is called for if any group which has been surveyed fails to meet the following criteria: Blood lead shall be no more than 20 μg/dl in 50% of the group; no more than 30 μg/dl in 90% and no more than 35 μg/dl in 98%. As has been mentioned earlier the results of the 1979 surveys in the United Kingdom are given in Appendix 2; it will be seen that the EEC criteria are easily met in most situations. Exceptions are a survey in Glasgow, where lead in tap water is known to be a problem, and three out of sixteen surveys related to lead industries. Remedial action is in hand in all these cases. As already noted, the criteria are well met amongst children living close to motorways and road junctions.

126 Our study of the effects of the different sources of lead has been handicapped by the lack of information simultaneously on blood lead and on exposure to lead from each of the major sources in a defined population. While it is likely that lead from one source affects the net retention of lead from another, there is no actual evidence that this occurs at the levels of source lead or blood lead found in the general environment and the general population. At present it is safe only to assume that summation will occur to a considerable degree.

127 The last 3 paragraphs have been concerned with the impact of representative levels of environmental lead upon the health of representative groups of people. They have dealt essentially with averages, with the advantages and disadvantages that the term implies. Exceptions are well known to occur. Variations both in the biological response to lead and in exposure are known to result in individual cases where the blood lead concentration is raised to levels meriting clinical concern. Effects on health that are judged to be lead-related may, however, not correspond to the observed blood lead concentration; sometimes there is an unusually high or low response of the blood lead concentration to a given exposure to lead. Most critically, of course, individual blood lead concentrations are affected by many external factors and notably by variations in environmental lead and by exposures to lead which are specific to the individual or the immediate locality. In the recent surveys carried out in collaboration with the EEC individuals with blood lead concentrations meriting clinical concern were specially looked for but only a few were found. The Working Party regard this as reassuring although not grounds for complacency as the EEC surveys did not examine small localised 'hot spots' where only a few people are exposed to higher than usual amounts of lead.

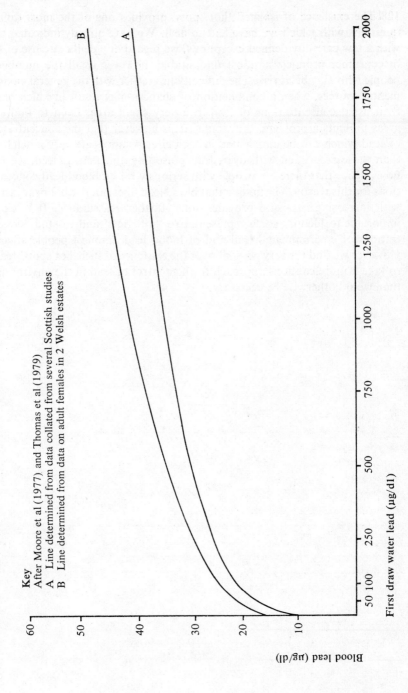

Figure 2: Relation of blood lead to first draw water lead

Key
After Moore et al (1977) and Thomas et al (1979)
A   Line determined from data collated from several Scottish studies
B   Line determined from data on adult females in 2 Welsh estates

First draw water lead (µg/dl)

Blood lead (µg/dl)

57

128 The existence of isolated 'hot spots' provides one of the most difficult questions with which we have had to deal. We have already indicated that, with a few carefully defined exceptions, we regard any deliberate use of lead in consumer products as most undesirable, however small the number of people who may be at risk. The difficulty lies rather with the general environmental sources, when a combination of chances may result in much higher than usual concentrations of lead in a very small area. Even to find such areas presents a problem. We would stress however that the concentrations of lead which can be anticipated in such circumstances are very much lower than those associated with overt lead poisoning and that, indeed, we have no evidence that there are people with seriously raised blood lead concentrations for this reason. The finding that blood lead does not rise in linear fashion with increasing exposure provides some further reassurance. It is clearly important to identify some representative 'hot spots' and to study concentrations of environmental lead and of blood lead amongst people affected. However we find the very possibility of the existence of such 'hot spots' reason to take a more cautious approach to the control of lead in the environment than would otherwise be necessary.

7 Neuropsychological Effects on Children

129 There is no doubt that lead is a toxic substance which in sufficient amounts can cause an encephalopathy which could result in permanent brain damage to babies and children. The response of a particular child exposed to lead from any source depends upon so intricate a network of inter-related factors that a simple relationship between dosage and degree of injury which would allow the relative risks to be calculated has not and possibly cannot be established. As with all biological phenomena, the sensitivity of any individual child to lead exposure will vary; nevertheless it is recognised that once a child shows signs of lead encephalopathy there is a danger that permanent damage may result.

130 A large proportion of the Working Party's time was devoted to the consideration of the effect of lead on the intelligence, behaviour, attainment and performance of children. Particular attention was given, therefore, to the possibility that exposure to lead at levels below those producing symptoms of poisoning can result in impaired intellectual functioning and related problems.

Problems of Analysis and Interpretation

Measurements

131 The total body burden of lead is divided among 3 compartments: (i) lead in blood and some soft tissues, which form a rapidly exchangeable pool; (ii) lead in soft tissue and loosely bound to bone, also rapidly exchangeable; and (iii) lead tightly bound in the skeleton, which comprises the major body burden. Although the determination of the concentration of lead in blood has limitations, it does give an indication of the amount of lead circulating in the blood at any one time. As has been explained earlier (paragraph 93) it is generally considered the most reliable biochemical index of recent lead exposure particularly in relation to environmental sources. The determination itself requires skill and meticulous attention to detail if inaccurate and imprecise results are to be avoided, especially at low concentrations

blood lead. At a value of 15 μg lead per dl blood the analyst should achieve a result within ±10% provided the quality control is meticulous. Many publications give no indication of accuracy and precision, making it impossible to assess the significance of the findings. Independent quality control schemes are essential to maintain standards of analysis. Results found in such schemes indicate that satisfactory accuracy and precision are not always obtained.

132 Since determinations on bone, which would be the best indicator of long-term exposure, are not feasible, some studies have been made on shed or extracted teeth of children. The determination of tooth lead is more complex than that of blood lead. Moreover, concentration appears to be higher in incisors than in molars and dentine is reported (Shapiro et al, 1972) to have an increased concentration of lead compared with that of enamel. In some studies the whole tooth is analysed, in others the crown and in some lead is determined in the individual tissues of the tooth. Note should be taken of these variables when comparing different sets of data. Accuracy and precision and the reproducibility of methods for separating dentine are exceedingly important in these determinations.

133 Some work has been performed on hair lead (Pihl & Parkes, 1977). This material presents problems with respect to the removal of surface contamination without extracting lead from the hair itself (paragraph 93). Hair is also affected by cosmetic treatments and samples of hair must be taken from identical parts of the scalp and an identical part of the length of the hair. Lead concentration in hair is not such a good indicator as blood of recent exposure, or as teeth as a measure of long-term exposure.

134 The Working Party was hampered surprisingly often by the omission of necessary data from published papers and in several cases direct approaches were made to the authors to obtain supplementary information. Published findings were assessed as far as possible in a standard manner, checking carefully such specific matters as the sampling and analytical methods used in the determination of lead in the environment, blood, teeth or other tissues, the types of tests used to study intellectual and behavioural development in children and the way in which the studies were designed and conducted. As a result it became apparent that there are critical defects in large parts of the evidence. Correct epidemiological methods are essential in such work; the selection of an appropriate population for study, the choice of controls and the need to obtain results from a sufficient proportion of those selected for study, are examples of points which are vital if valid results are to be obtained but which are often neglected in the work which we have reviewed. At the same time we emphasise that the subject is inherently difficult. Variations in

intelligence and behaviour are associated with many social, genetic and environmental factors, which must be taken into account in any study which hopes to distinguish any effects of lead. Intelligence, behaviour and the interfering factors are very difficult to measure reliably. A point which requires emphasis is that association does not necessarily imply causation; in order to judge the confidence with which cause-and-effect relationships could be inferred from the studies as a whole, we used the requirements set out originally by Sir Austin Bradford Hill and which are reproduced in Appendix 3.

135 There are difficulties in obtaining sensitive and valid measures of children's intellectual and behavioural functioning, especially if group tests have to be applied to samples of the general population. Tests used vary from rather crude screening to detailed individual testing of a wide range of skills. The former will not only constitute less valid reflections of intelligence, but will also be more likely to miss deficits which are restricted to certain specific types of intellectual functioning. For most standard tests the child has only to sustain his attention and performance over limited periods. Consequently the tests tend to be insensitive to deficits which concern the child's ability to organise his work and to sustain application and attention over long periods when unsupervised.

136 The results of most intelligence tests are expressed as an Intelligent Quotient (IQ) which is standardized for age to give a mean of 100 points with a standard deviation of 15 points. Where the tests are carried out by several examiners, the variation can sometimes be very large unless testers are well trained. However, the most likely source of bias can be the examiner's prior knowledge of the child's lead levels, for where assessments have not been 'blind' there is always the possibility that any differences found may have been an artefact resulting from the examiner's expectations.

137 The problems concerned with the measurement of behavioural disorders are discussed later in this chapter. It is desirable to carry out the observations on eg activity level, in at least two situations as the assessments made at home and at school only correlate weakly.

Effect of Social Conditions on the Measurements

138 One of the major problems in both analysing and interpreting studies of this type is that of confounding variables. Exposure to lead tends to be associated with poor environmental conditions, eg old houses with lead-

containing paintwork, houses close to sources of lead emission, such as smelter or battery works, or to roads with high traffic density. In general, children with lower than average intelligence tend to come from families living in areas where the standard of nutrition and schooling may be low and where their companions are affected by the same depressed environment. Often such areas are in the inner part of a city where the exposure to lead is also greatest.

139 For example, descriptions of the living conditions of the children from areas close to lead smelter works at the time of some of the studies considered illustrate the type of social problems which can occur. In the first the description is of Mexican Americans living in the community of Smeltertown, El Paso. 'Smeltertown was a small (0.1 km × 0.5 km) community isolated by the Rio Grande River and a large lead smelter. The area contained no drainage system, no municipal sewage system, no grass and essentially no traffic. Annual precipitation is 6–8 inches a year, but approximately half of this comes in one or two storms during the summer. The earthen yards and streets provided a convenient playground for year-round out-door activity. We identified 206 children living in this area' (McNeil et al, 1975). The second written by a journalist in 1972 refers to the Isle of Dogs in England. '. . . A Desperate Place . . . Every indication of urban health is pointing resolutely downward. The housing is mostly unattractive and unpopulated. . . . At one stage there were 400 Council flats untaken. It is hard to see why any young people should stay'.

140 However, although the same terms are used in the USA, UK and other countries to describe variables such as poor housing or social class, social patterns may differ widely so that their effect cannot be easily translated from one country to another or even from one study to another.

Effect of Medical Conditions on the Measurements

141 As well as the confounding variables due to social conditions there are many medical conditions which can have a depressing effect, both permanent and transitory, on the child's response to an IQ test. Babies who have suffered various forms of birth injury and anoxia, as well as children who have brain damage from an infection or an accident may well have a permanent IQ deficit ranging from slight to gross. Although it is normal practice to exclude these children from the analysis, it is not always done. Minor degrees of ill-health, such as an infection, anaemia or poor nutrition, may cause a temporary lack of responsiveness. While motivation is usually included as part of the general psychological assessment of the child, most studies rely on a single

IQ measurement so that no allowance is made for any temporary upset in the child. Children who are mentally retarded may take longer to learn to walk and may therefore be exposed to lead-containing dust and dirt for a longer period than those who are mobile earlier, as well as being more likely to have abnormal habits, such as eating paint, plaster and dirt. Thus, they run the risk of having a higher than average intake of lead.

Terminology

142 Several terms used in the studies have different meanings in the USA and the UK or are not precisely defined and are difficult to interpret.

(a) Asymptomatic lead poisoning: The symptoms which suggest early lead intoxication are apathy, loss of appetite, anaemia and abdominal pain. Convulsions, ataxia, persistent vomiting and coma denote the onset of encephalopathy. The terms clinical, subclinical, asymptomatic and symptomatic are used to distinguish the cases clinically, but they are often not precisely defined. This means that whereas cases with lead encephalopathy will be called clinical or symptomatic, it is not always clear into which group patients with symptoms or signs of lead poisoning not involving the central nervous system are assigned. (b) Pica: This term is used loosely in the literature and is usually defined as the ingestion of non-food materials such as paint and dirt and is described in more detail in Chapter 5. The same word is sometimes used to describe 'mouthing' where the material is not ingested. The term is used differently by various authors. (c) Hyperactivity: The term is used differently in the USA from the UK. This subject is discussed in more detail later in this chapter.

Selection of Cases for Study

143 Population studies carried out in the UK have shown that the proportion of children with raised lead levels is small. With the increasing use of more sophisticated psychological tests which are time consuming and expensive, the number so examined has to be restricted and as it is rarely possible to include all children, some form of sampling has to be carried out.

144 In many studies the concentration at which the blood lead is called 'raised' is prejudged; usually around 30 or 40 $\mu g/dl$. A child with a blood lead above this is then matched with another child whose blood lead is below this level. Because there is no top limit the 'raised' blood lead concentrations can

have a wide range. Nevertheless if a deficit in the IQs is found, the prejudged cut off point is often taken as the threshold level above which the lead in the blood can have a deleterious effect, although this may not be so. In interpreting these findings it is important to bear in mind that the number of children with the higher blood lead concentrations is usually very small and the results in this group can vary considerably. The results of matched control studies cannot reveal directly a dose response relationship; only studies sampling across the total population can do so.

145 The greatest problem, however, lies in the selection of children for comparison. The majority of studies attempt to find matched controls but with so large a number of variables the matching has to be limited and it is rare to take more than one control. In some cases no attempt has been made to match the groups and statistical methods, eg multivariate analysis, are used to assess the relative contributions made by various factors to explain the associations observed. Unfortunately, full details of the methods used are often omitted from the published reports. Most statistical tests are applicable to a normal distribution but that of blood lead values is skewed. The use of inappropriate methods of analysis will therefore result in problems of interpretation.

Effects of Lead on Intellectual Function

146 Different issues arise in connection with different types of investigation. These are discussed under the following headings: clinic-type studies; studies of mentally retarded children; smelter studies; and general population studies of dental lead.

Clinic-type studies of children with high lead levels

147 Under this heading the following studies were considered: De la Burde and Choate (1972, 1975); Perino and Ernhart (1974); Kotok (1972); Kotok *et al* (1977); Rummo *et al* (1979); Baloh *et al* (1975); Needleman (1977); Albert *et al* (1974); Sachs *et al* (1978, 1979); Pueschel *et al* (1972). Some of these studies report on patients who have received treatment with chelating agents to reduce the blood lead concentration. All these studies were carried out over a period of seven years during which time there has been a considerable accumulation of knowledge. The findings tend to be contradictory; some studies claim that persistently raised lead levels above 60 $\mu g/dl$ can be associated with a reduction in performance in intelligence tests among

even asymptomatic children; on the other hand, other studies do not claim to show this relationship. Greater decrements and associated behavioural disorders are evident in children who have suffered from lead encephalopathy.

Studies of mentally retarded children

148 Under this heading the following studies were considered: David *et al* (1976a, 1978); Moncrieff *et al* (1964); Gibson *et al* (1967); Youroukos *et al* (1978); Beattie *et al* (1975); Moore *et al* (1977b). Imperfect methods were used in all of these studies which makes it difficult to draw any conclusions (Rutter, 1980). The findings are sufficient to mark these out as potential risk groups for increased lead exposure but it remains uncertain how far the raised lead levels are a cause or effect of the mental retardation.

Smelter studies

149 Under this heading the following studies were considered: Lansdown *et al* (1974); Landrigan *et al* (1975a & b); Whitworth *et al* (1974); McNeil *et al* (1975); Hebel *et al* (1976); Ratcliffe (1977); Wegner (1976); Gregory *et al* (1976). As noted, studies of children living nearby compared with those far away from an extrinsic source of lead should constitute a good test of the hypothesis that raised lead levels cause intellectual deficits or behavioural deviance. In fact this has not proved to be the case, in part because very large samples are needed to test for small differences and in part because of incomplete reporting and inadequate analyses of some of the studies undertaken. Some of the studies report a mean IQ deficit of up to 5 points associated with raised lead concentrations in an approximate range of 40–80 μg/dl. However, other studies with equally high blood levels do not show this relationship.

General population studies of dental lead

150 Several general population studies of dental lead published in the last few years have suggested that modest exposure to environmental lead may be causally related to intellectual deficits in children. In view of the importance and implications of this suggestion, a fuller discussion of the relevant studies will be included in this section.

151 Needleman and Shapiro (1974) reported that dentine lead levels are higher in children with lead poisoning than in asymptomatic children; similar

65

results have been obtained by De la Burde and Choate (1975). It is also known that dentine lead is higher in a school district in Philadelphia in which there was a high concentration of smelters, foundries and lead processing plants than in a district without these industrial activities (Needleman et al, 1974) and this difference has been attributed to airborne lead.

152 A more recent study (Needleman et al, 1979) has investigated the neuropsychological functioning of children in the general population with 'high' and 'low' levels as assessed by dentine analysis using shed deciduous teeth from first and second grade children in two towns in Massachusetts between 1975 and 1978. Of 3,329 children, 2,235 donated one or more teeth and the teachers completed a behavioural assessment questionnaire on 2,146 of these children. The mean lead level of the teeth was 14 ppm (μg/g) with a Standard Deviation of 9 (Needleman et al, 1979). The analysis was repeated for those in the highest 10th centile (greater than 24 μg/g) and in the lowest 10th centile (less than 6 μg/g). If the concordant samples gave a mean level of greater than 20 μg/g or lower than 10 μg/g they were classified as 'high' and 'low' lead respectively and the remainder were called unclassified. This gave a total of 524 subjects of whom 254 were excluded because of 'bilingual homes, not interested, moved, infant at home, two working parents etc'; the remaining 270 children were tested but of a further 112, 76 children 'whose birthweight was below 2,500g, who were not discharged at the same time as their mother after birth, or who had a history of noteworthy head injury and any child who had been diagnosed as lead-poisoned' were excluded; the remaining 36 were excluded because the later tooth analysis was discordant. The final sample for statistical analysis was 158, ie 100 'low' and 58 'high' lead.

153 Detailed neuropsychological testing was then carried out in the children of both groups while the mothers completed social and medical questionnaires and tests to assess attitude and vocabulary. In addition, the teachers completed an 11-item forced-choice behavioural rating on each child. The choice of the tests was generally sound. The high and low lead groups were broadly similar on background variables but the high lead group was slightly older, slightly more socially disadvantaged and the parental IQ's were slightly lower. Variables other than pica, which differentiated the two groups, were used throughout the analyses as covariates. The validity of the high-low dentine lead differentiation was tested through the association with blood lead levels estimated 4–5 years earlier in approximately half of the children. The high lead group had had a mean blood lead level of 35.5 μg/dl (range 18–54) compared with 23.8 μg/dl (range 12–37) for the low lead group. Unfortunately, no analyses of the children's behaviour or educational attainment were under taken in relation to these blood levels.

154 After an analysis of covariance, the corrected mean full scale WISC-R IQ of the low dentine group was 106.6 compared with 102.1 for the high lead children (p = 0.03). Examination of the individual subtest scores and of the various additional tests showed a general tendency for the high lead children to perform less well. The authors state that verbal performance and auditory processing was particularly impaired but the variations between different types of test functions were quite small. The findings are highly suggestive but some caution is needed in their interpretation. Several questions were left unanswered in the published paper (Needleman et al, 1979) but some were adequately dealt with in personal communication. For example, the dentine lead levels reported, are quite different from those of Hrdina and Winneke (1978), and De la Burde and Choate (1975). This may be due to methodological differences in sampling dentine lead; a possible source of bias lies in the effect of caries or fillings since both are associated with social variables. However, since less than 1 % of teeth were discarded for this reason it seems unlikely that this had any appreciable effect on the results.

155 A further limitation in the published paper is the fact that pica was not used as a covariate although the high lead children had a much higher frequency of this condition (29 % cf 11 %). Although pica was not associated with the behavioural ratings it was associated with performance IQ in both the low and the high tooth lead group and with verbal IQ in the low lead but not the high lead group. The possibility remains that both pica and raised lead levels are independently associated with lower IQ. Another question concerns the effect of omitting the middle group of children with dentine lead levels between 8.5 and 20. It seems important to know whether the intermediate lead group was also psychologically intermediate; if it were not it would weaken the argument that the association represents a causal influence of lead. Furthermore, it is not known how much bias has been created by the very high non-cooperation rate.

156 These data also raise the broader question of how the high lead group had come to have a higher body lead burden and also the adequacy of the control of the family variables which relied on relatively crude and incomplete questionnaire data. Two further uncertainties arise in the comparison of the results of the Needleman study with those of other investigators. Firstly, his findings are strongest with respect to behaviour whereas in other studies the associations between raised lead levels and behaviour disturbances have been both weaker and less consistent than those with impaired intelligence. Secondly, the findings of a 4-point IQ difference in the means with respect to dentine lead levels equivalent to the difference of mean blood lead of 35.5 to 23.8 μg/dl suggests that a very much greater IQ difference should be associated

with blood lead concentrations in the range 40–80 μg/dl. However, this has not been shown in any studies and IQ differences associated with high blood lead concentrations in asymptomatic children have also been in the 4 to 5 points range, which implies a mechanism very different from that with respect to other biological hazards to the brain, eg head injury.

157 It must be emphasised that many of the queries raised here apply even more strongly to most other investigations but the Needleman study has been discussed in detail because it is one of the most comprehensive so far undertaken. The implication of the findings is that children in roughly the top 10% of the dentine lead distribution as defined in this study differ from those in the bottom 10% in intelligence and the mean difference in the intelligence quotient is of the order of 4 points after correcting for differences in family background. It is suggested that the 4 point mean difference in the two groups is associated with a difference in mean blood lead concentrations between 23 and 35 μg/dl although this is based on blood lead determinations performed some 4–5 years previously on approximately half of the children involved in the study.

158 There is an urgent need for independent replication of the above study and in this connection that of Hrdina and Winneke (1978) appears particularly crucial. The basic design, ie studying extreme groups was similar. Incisor teeth were collected from 458 seven to ten year old children in the German city of Duisberg. Twenty-six children with a dentine lead below 3 μg/g (mean 2.4) were compared with 26 with a level exceeding 7 (mean 9.2); the groups being matched on age, sex and father's occupation. The response rate differed between the groups (77% control and 61% high lead). The two groups did not differ significantly in background characteristics but the high lead group showed more perinatal risk factors. The high lead group had a mean IQ level some 5 to 7 points below controls but the difference fell short of statistical significance. The results of the study are generally in keeping with those of Needleman et al (1979) but unfortunately the numbers were small and the group differences were not controlled for background factors. The queries raised with respect to the Needleman et al (1979) study also apply in this case. It should also be noted that the dentine lead levels in this study were lower than those of Needleman et al (1979) (the mean of 9.2 μg/g in the high lead group was less than half the lower cut-off of 20 used in the latter study).

159 Together these studies (Needleman et al, 1979; Hrdina and Winneke, 1978) provide some evidence of an association between raised tooth dentine lead levels and a slight lowering of measured intelligence. There are a number

of reservations about these studies and the inferences to be drawn from them which in our view weakens their conclusions.

Effects of Lead on Educational Attainment and Behaviour

160 In an earlier study on children with lead poisoning (Byers and Lord, 1943) most of the children showed poor school performance after lead intoxication but the absence of either controls or pre-poisoning measurements makes it impossible to determine how far the psychological deficits were directly due to the lead intoxication. Following these findings concern has been expressed that exposure to lead has adverse effects on children's psychological development. However it should be noted that methods of treatment have now improved considerably. In recent years the hypothesis has been proposed that lower levels of lead absorption than those leading to lead intoxication may be associated with an increase in learning difficulties and behavioural problems. In particular, it has been claimed that increased blood lead concentrations are associated with hyperactivity. This section will examine the evidence in relation to associations with children's behaviour in three areas: (i) educational attainment; (ii) hyperactivity and (iii) other behavioural disorders.

(i) *Educational attainment*

161 Although widespread concern has been expressed that raised blood lead concentrations are associated with poor educational attainment, sound evidence on the strength and nature of such an association is lacking. Some studies have relied on global ratings made by teachers or parents, often after the lead level is known and little attention has been paid to the intricacies of measuring educational attainment. Two main conceptual distinctions need to be recognised. Firstly, poor educational attainment is clearly related to a wide range of indices of social disadvantage (Rutter *et al*, 1970b). Since such measures also appear to be related to higher blood lead concentrations it is necessary to demonstrate statistically that lead and attainment are still related after the influence of mediating social factors has been taken into account. Secondly, it is recognised that *backwardness* in attainment must be differentiated from *underachievement* (Rutter and Yule, 1975). Whilst it would be of concern to find that children with relatively high blood lead concentrations tended to score at lower levels than their peers on standardised tests of reading, mathematics, spelling or other tests of educational attainment, it would be of equal concern to discover that they were underachieving in the

sense of doing less well than expected on the basis of their measured intelligence. To date, no study has used adequate measures of intelligence and attainment to allow such questions to be answered.

162 Albert et al (1974) reported an increase in special class placements in schools in children with symptoms of lead poisoning other than encephalopathy (19%) and in children with blood levels above 60 μg/dl (9%) compared with a control group (3%). However, the children's attainment was not measured and the groups were not matched for socio-economic variables. Pihl and Parkes (1977) attempted to examine the association the other way round. They compared the hair lead levels of 31 'learning disabled' children with 22 controls. Unfortunately, their definition of 'learning disability' is unacceptable psychometrically, so that their findings of higher levels of many elements, including lead, is of doubtful validity. Lansdown et al (1974) gathered data on children's intelligence and reading levels, but did not publish the latter results. However, they found no relationship between blood lead levels and scores on a word reading test. (Lansdown, personal communication).

163 Hebel et al (1976) report a tendency, although not statistically significant, for children living closer to a battery factory in Birmingham to score about 1 or 2 points lower on verbal reasoning, mathematics and English than those living further away. The differences remained after adjusting for social class, birth rank and maternal age. However, since the children's blood lead levels were not taken it is difficult to relate these findings to actual, as opposed to assumed, lead exposure. Needleman et al (1979) assessed the children's educational attainment but do not report their results.

(ii) *Hyperactivity*

164 Although it appears to be widely held that an association has been demonstrated between high body lead levels and hyperactivity in children, there is no satisfactory evidence which confirms this view. It is clear that American writers use the terms 'hyperactivity' and 'hyperkinesis' much more loosely than clinicians in Britain (Sandberg et al, 1978). Recent evidence suggests that children's levels of activity must be monitored in at least two different settings before a diagnosis of hyperactivity can be considered. Moreover, few of the existing rating scales stand close psychometric scrutiny.

165 The main papers which relate to this question are summarised below. Baloh et al (1975) compared 27 high lead children with a similar number of

low lead children. While the two groups did not differ on a number of indices such as IQ scores and did not differ on their level of activity during testing, nevertheless, 44% of the high lead children compared with 15% of the controls were regarded as 'hyperactive' by either parents or teachers. It is unfortunate that standardised questionnaires were not used since this markedly reduces the weight that can be given to this isolated finding. Landrigan et al (1975 a & b) found no differences between high lead groups and controls on hyperactivity whether measured by parental questionnaire or as observed by a physician. McNeil et al (1975) used the Werry–Weiss–Peters hyperactivity scale and found no difference between high lead children and controls. Needleman et al (1979) asked teachers of over 2,300 children to complete an unstandardised, crude rating scale of 11 simple yes-no items. Nine of the items showed increasing 'pathology' with increasing tooth lead levels. One of the items which failed to show such a relationship was 'hyperactive'. David et al (1972, 1976b, 1977) studied hyperactive children and claimed that they had higher levels of lead in their blood. However, his definition of hyperactivity in this study is dubious and the methodology is such that no firm conclusions can be drawn from his work.

(iii) *Other behavioural disorders*

166 What is really at issue is whether small increases of lead in the body cause subtle alterations to the functioning of the central nervous system (CNS). Unfortunately, only the grossest changes in CNS functioning can, at present, be reliably detected (Rutter et al, 1970a). Attributes which have long been regarded as associated with CNS dysfunction, such as disturbances in attention span, distractibility, poor learning, etc, cannot be readily measured. Certainly they cannot be adequately measured by rating scales completed by parents and teachers. It is possible to make some assessments using time-consuming individual testing in laboratories. To date such studies are rarely done with any groups of children and so it is not surprising to find few good studies of children with high body lead burdens.

167 Following work with adult patients affected by very high lead doses, some studies have investigated children's reaction times. Needleman (1977) reports a significantly slowed reaction time in his high lead group. Landrigan et al (1975 a & b) reported that their high level group were significantly slower in a wrist-tapping test. Rummo (1974) reports that high lead concentrations were associated with slowed reaction times, slower wrist-tapping and poor leg coordination. The effects were most marked at very high lead levels, but trends were also evident at more modest levels. Baloh et al (1975) found that

their high lead group did less well on tests of fine motor ability, although the difference was not statistically significant. Two studies report on the results applying the Frostig Test of Developmental Perception; Needleman (1977) found significantly lower scores on eye-hand coordination, but Ratcliffe (1977) reported only small and non-significant differences between her groups. This discrepancy may reflect little more than the crudeness of the tests used. De la Burde and Choate (1972) found that their high lead group contained 32% with reportedly short attention spans compared with only 14% in their control group. Only one other study appears to have commented on this directly. Needleman *et al* (1979) report near-linear relationships between tooth lead level and distractibility, lack of persistence, impulsivity and day-dreaming. Unfortunately the rating scale items were not standardised and social and other factors were not taken into account.

168 In summary it can be stated that up to the present no study has satis-factorily demonstrated a relationship between increasing body lead burden and either educational attainment or hyperactivity. Measuring subtle effects requires sophisticated techniques and these have not so far been employed. There are far fewer data on all aspects of behaviour and adjustment other than intelligence. There are a few indications that reaction times and fine motor coordination may be impaired at high lead levels, but it must be stressed that these are very tentative findings.

Epidemiological Aspects of the Papers on the Effect of Exposure to Lead on the Mental Development of Children

169 The object of this section has been to devise a framework which would enable the results from several studies on the effect of exposure to lead on the mental development of children to be compared with each other. Sixteen published papers were found which would allow such a comparison. The studies were of three types:—

(a) *Effect of pollution from smelters or lead battery works.* There were five in all. Two compared the children with blood levels of over 40 μg/dl with matched controls who had levels of less than 40 μg/dl (Landrigan *et al*, 1975b; Gregory *et al*, 1976). One had a complicated structured sample comparing children with different blood lead levels (Ratcliffe, 1977). The remaining two compared populations living at varying distances from the smelter (Lansdown *et al*, 1974; McNeil *et al*, 1975).

(b) *Population studies.* In two cohort studies, the children had been followed up since birth and, from information already gathered, groups were defined and compared with matched controls from the same cohort (De la Burde and Choate, 1972, 1975). There were three studies where the children had been selected from a school population who had donated teeth. Those whose teeth had a high lead content were matched with others with a low lead content (Hrdina and Winneke, 1978) or the group with the highest tooth lead was compared with another group with the lowest tooth lead, but they were not matched (Needleman *et al*, 1978, 1979).

(c) *Hospital studies.* In these five studies, selected hospital patients with a history of exposure to lead were compared with a control group. In the first patients were matched with their siblings (Sachs *et al*, 1978). In three studies patients with varying degrees of lead intoxication were matched with controls (Albert *et al*, 1974; Kotok *et al*, 1977; Rummo *et al*, 1979). In the fifth, patients with blood lead levels greater than 50 $\mu g/dl$ were matched with patients with a level of less than 30 $\mu g/dl$ (Baloh *et al*, 1975).

Measurements

170 To compare the results it was assumed that the deficit between two IQ means using the same standardised scale could be compared with the deficit between two IQ means using another standardised scale, regardless of the age of the children. While it is possible that these differences are not strictly comparable, it is unlikely to have any appreciable effect upon the results and the conclusions drawn from this analysis. Unfortunately, the lead levels were not so easy to compare, as different methods were used to identify the high and low lead groups. In some cases the blood analysis had been carried out several years before the IQ tests. Where the blood tests had been repeated when the IQ tests were carried out, those nearest in time were used in the analysis. Sometimes mean levels were not given, merely the cut-off points, eg above and below 30 $\mu g/dl$ blood lead. In some the mean related to a wide range of observations, while in others the distibution was curtailed. Therefore, the differences between the mean IQs and the mean blood levels could not be compared in all the studies. A major difficulty which is inherent in any combination of studies is that the results of investigations of a very different quality have to be pooled.

171 The studies were first ordered according to the differences in the mean IQs between the high and low lead groups and according to the type of study. Two of the hospital studies included different groups of patients, compared with a single control and these were separated so that each group could be compared with the control. There were, therefore, 20 items among the 16 studies.

172 The comparison is presented in Table 14 and diagramatically in Figure 3. Along the base of the figure are the number of studies according to the differences in mean IQ and above each study is the highest and lowest mean blood lead level (where known). It can be seen that there is little relationship between the size of the difference between the mean blood lead concentrations and the mean IQ differences. However, there is an ordering of the studies. The results from the hospitals spread from no effect to a large deficit in IQ. Those from the smelter studies range from no loss to a deficit of 5 points and those from the population studies a deficit of 4 up to 10 points. All three types overlap around the 5 point mark resulting in a clustering of the observations.

173 Both of the smelter studies where no loss of IQ was noted were concerned with the proximity of the homes of the children to the smelter works. In the first the whole population was used. In the second those living close to the works were matched with children living further away. These were the only two independent studies which had similar designs; in both cases the blood tests were carried out two to four years before the IQ tests. One showed a deficit of 2 and the other of 5 points in the IQ. One study was different from the others because of the sampling method, the use of the Griffiths test, the young age of the children, the fact that the source of the lead was a battery works and that the blood samples were taken two years before the IQ test. In this study there was a deficit of 5 points IQ.

174 Only two population studies recorded the blood lead measurements and the differences between the means were the smallest among all the papers. These two and one other study did not use matched controls and relied on later statistical analysis to correct for any bias. On the other hand in the study with the smallest IQ deficit, the children who had pica for paint were matched with others in the cohort who did not; unfortunately blood lead measurements were not given but the differences between the mean tooth lead levels were large (202 and 112 μg/g).

175 In the hospital studies the criteria for selecting the index cases were usually more carefully defined than in the other studies. All were compared with controls and, where the blood lead concentrations were known, the mean differences were greater. The largest deficit in IQs occurred in those children with symptoms and there was little or no deficit where the differences in the mean blood lead concentrations were small. Intermediate deficits occur but it is difficult to draw conclusions from them since they are associated with wide ranges of blood lead concentrations, not all are controlled for pica and there is wide variation in the duration of exposure.

176 The hospital studies suggest that the presence of lead encephalopathy can result in an overall lowering of the IQ of the children, but the extent of the deficit is difficult to quantify and may even be relatively small if the family background and improved treatment over the years is taken into account. They do also suggest that only minor effects can be demonstrated despite quite high blood lead levels if the patients are asymptomatic. However, hospital patients are a highly selected group and studies based on their experience and extrapolated to the community as a whole can be misleading.

177 Logically it might be expected that the children living close to smelter works would be exposed to the same hazards as the population as a whole as well as the emissions from the works so that their blood lead levels would be higher than those in the population studies. With one exception this is true. In one study the control group had a slightly lower mean blood lead level than that of the low lead groups from the population studies, but in this case the control group was taken from children living some distance from the works. All the high levels were much greater than those of the population studies and, therefore, the differences between the blood means were much greater. But, contrary to expectations, the IQ deficits were generally less than those found among the population studies.

178 This review has shown that the deficits in IQs noted in the various studies show little relationship with the size of the difference in the mean blood lead levels. It suggests that the selection of the control group is of crucial importance and it may be that factors other than the exposure to lead may have a more direct bearing on the IQ differences. In addition, several of the studies suffer seriously from a large loss of cases, which could introduce serious bias and from inadequate matching. It should also be noted that in most of the studies there is inadequate description of the main source of lead, its chemical and physical form, the length of exposure or the dosage.

Table 14 Studies ordered according to the type of study and the difference in mean IQs

Study No.	Difference in IQ	Test	Difference in mean Blood Lead	Range Blood Lead High	Range Blood Lead Low
Smelter Studies					
1	+ †	W	—	—	—
2	+ 1	W	30	14–93	7–43
3	− 2	W	26‡	—	—
4	− 5	W	14‡	22–58	15–39
5	− 5	G	16♦	36–74	18–35
Population Studies					
6	− 4	W	Tooth	—	—
7	− 5	W	Tooth (Blood 12)	Top blood level (54.0)	
8	− 5	SB	—	—	—
9	− 7	W	Tooth (Blood 11)	(18–54) Blood	(12–37) Blood
10	− 7	W(H)	Tooth	—	—
11	−10	Mc	—	40–70	10–30
Hospital Studies					
12	+ 5	W	Tooth ♦	—	—
13	+ 2	W	—	50–365	<40
14	+ 1	Mc	25	Max 61	Max 23
12	+ 1	W	Tooth ♦	—	—
15	− 1	W	20‡	13–69	13–39
16	*	—	51	61–200	11–40
14	− 6	Mc	30	Max 68	Max 23
12	−12	W	Tooth ♦	—	—
14	−17	Mc	37	Max 88	Max 23

Footnotes

All blood leads are expressed as μg/dl.

‡Sampled from results of an earlier blood test. The mean concentration is that at the time of the IQ.

♦Blood lead levels taken some years before the test.

( )The figures in brackets are differences in mean blood lead concentration (taken 4–5 years previously) the primary measure being difference in tooth lead.

†A series of different measurements given. All mean IQ results higher in high lead group.

*A series of cognitive measurements given but no formal IQ tests performed. The differences in IQ equivalents varied from −1 to −9. No significant differences in classes evaluated.

IQ Tests: W = WISC   SB = Stanford Binet   W(H) = WISC
   Mc = McCarthy   G = Griffiths   (Hamburg Weschler Intelligence test for Children)

Total population.
Living close to smelter matched with those away.
>40 matched with <40.
>40 matched with <40.
>35 and <35 structured sample. Battery works.

Pica with paint v controls. From known cohort.
Selected from lowest and highest tenth centile.
Not matched.
Pica with paint plus those with raised blood lead v controls. From known cohort – no
blood lead measurements.
Tooth <8.5 compared with >20. Not matched.

High tooth (mean 9.2) matched with low (mean 2.4).
Inner city population. Not matched.

Blood lead <60 both groups. Tooth high in one.
Patients v siblings.
Short exposure v controls.
Blood >60 asymptomatic v <60.
>50 v <30 at earlier test.
Pts. v controls. Matched for pica.
Long exposure v controls.
Blood >60 symptomatic v <60.
Encephalopathy v controls.

References
Study
No
 1   Lansdown, R G *et al* (1974)
 2   McNeil, J L *et al* (1975)
 3   Gregory, R J *et al* (1976)
 4   Landrigan, P J *et al* (1975b)
 5   Ratcliffe, J M (1977)
 6   De La Burde, B & Choate M S (1975)
 7   Needleman, H L *et al* (1979)
 8   De La Burde, B & Choate, M S (1972)
 9   Needleman, H L *et al* (1978)
10   Hrdina, K & Winneke, G (1978)
11   Perino, J & Ernhart, C B (1974)
12   Albert, R E *et al* (1974)
13   Sachs, H K *et al* (1978)
14   Rummo, J H *et al* (1979)
15   Baloh, R *et al* (1975)
16   Kotok, D *et al* (1977)

Figure 3: Differences in mean IQ and mean blood lead in high and low lead groups

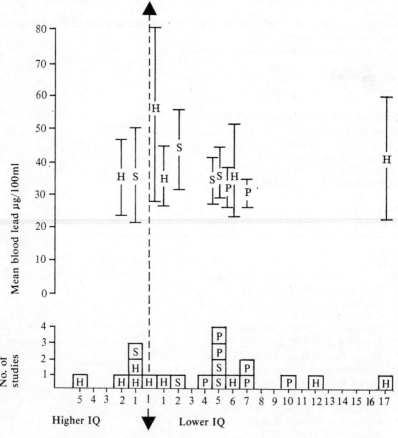

Key
High mean

Type of study (S, P or H)

S = Smelter
P = Population.
H = Hospital

Low mean

Differences in mean blood lead (where known)

Mean blood lead µg/100ml

No. of studies

Higher IQ   Lower IQ

Difference in general IQ between high and low lead groups

179 As already mentioned most of the surveys on the effect of exposure of lead on children have been carried out in countries other than the UK where social and educational conditions may be different. In the American studies where a group of children with 'raised lead' levels had been matched with a 'low lead' group for sex, social class and other variables, the mean IQs of the low lead control groups were below the population average of 100. For example, in the three American smelter studies (McNeil et al, 1975; Landrigan et al, 1975b; Gregory et al, 1976) the mean IQs of the matched controls were 89, 93 and 96 and in the hospital studies they were in the lower 90s or the upper 80s. It is only in the unmatched population studies that the mean IQs of the control groups were above 100. In the two American studies (Needleman et al 1978, 1979) they were 109 and 107 (WISC-R) and in the German study 130 (HAWIK) (Hrdina and Winneke, 1978).

180 No general population surveys have been carried out in this country. Three smelter type studies have been undertaken, but without matched controls as they were designed to demonstrate the effect of lead emitted from a single source and either all the affected population or a representative sample was examined. In one of these studies using WISC the children living close to the smelter had results which were marginally higher than those of the children living furthest away (Lansdown et al, 1974). In another, with assessments based on 11+ examination results, the children living close to a source of lead contamination (a battery works) had results which were virtually no different from those for children living further from the source (Hebel et al, 1976). In neither of these studies did the differences reach statistical significance. In the third (Ratcliffe, 1977) the general quotient was 108 (Griffiths) in the 'moderate' lead group and 102 (Griffiths) in the 'high' lead group; this difference was not statistically significant and an analysis of the various factors affecting the results showed that the variations in the developmental scores appeared to be related to age and attendance at primary school.

181 There have been several surveys of mentally handicapped children in the UK which have shown that mentally retarded children, on average, have higher blood lead levels than children who are not retarded (Moncrieff et al, 1964; Gibson et al, 1967; Moore et al, 1977b; Beattie et al, 1975). As already discussed, it is not possible to say from these studies whether the lead was a contributory cause of the mental handicap or vice versa. Thus, the few studies in the UK of asymptomatic children have not so far demonstrated a significant deficit in IQ due to exposure to lead and, in the light of the results

from the EEC survey (Appendix 2) the impression is gained that the proportion of children with a raised blood lead level might not be as great as that found in the USA (Morbidity & Mortality Weekly Report, 1979). However, the number of UK studies is very limited and the need for further research is again stressed.

8 Discussion and General Conclusions

182 The main body of our report gives a clear indication of the complexities of the issues that we have studied and the inconclusive nature of the evidence concerning adverse effects of small amounts of lead taken up gradually from environmental sources. Despite the appearance of several new and important reports on this topic during the course of our work, many uncertainties remain; there is still much difficulty in assessing the magnitude of any effects and in trying to disentangle the role of lead from that of many other relevant factors liable to affect mental development and behaviour. We have noted that several new studies are in progress, in this country as well as abroad, and we have put forward recommendations for further research. The problem is by no means resolved; while we hope that better designed studies will help to clarify some of the outstanding issues, we recognise that it will remain difficult to obtain clear-cut answers.

183 We have not considered it necessary to devote much time to the relatively well-understood question of lead poisoning. While there has been a reduction in the occurrence of such cases over the past few decades, we are concerned about the numbers that still occur. An attendant worry is that there may be additional cases that are not reported or that remain undiagnosed. By far the largest proportion of clinical cases of lead poisoning among children arise through pica (defined in paragraph 142), as has been described earlier in this report.

184 We have noted the requirements of the EEC regarding blood lead concentrations in the general population and the reference levels recommended by WHO. In the absence of clear findings relating blood lead concentrations encountered in the general population to defined effects on health we have not ourselves sought to give any guidance on threshold levels.

185 An important part of our work has been to identify the circumstances liable to result in elevated blood lead concentrations, particularly in children. Our comments are based on existing exposure levels in the United Kingdom

and we have seen that a great diversity of sources is involved. There is clear evidence that 'hot spots' occur and it must be asked whether the exposures involved are acceptable. Progress which is being made, eg in the elimination of special problems of contamination of tap water in some areas, is mentioned in the relevant sections below.

Lead in Food

186 Recent investigations, including monitoring and analysis of diets by MAFF, have shown clearly that most people in the UK derive the major part of their lead body burden from food. We have seen no evidence that conflicts with this conclusion. Part of the lead content of some foods comes from the air through direct contamination and from translocation from soil into vegetables and grasses. The contribution that this makes to the body burden needs further investigation.

187 The World Health Organisation has set international guidance criteria on permissible levels for lead in food. These are well above the usual maximum amounts that are found in food in the United Kingdom. However, we do not consider it satisfactory to rest on the assumption that because exposure to lead from food in the UK is below WHO limits, a satisfactory state of affairs necessarily exists. We also recognise that MAFF, with the cooperation of the food industry, has been grappling with this problem for some years and that there has been recent amending legislation limiting still further the lead content of food.

188 We have noted that canned foods are a well defined source of lead. Special attention to this point has been given by MAFF who, in conjunction with industry, has introduced specific measures to ensure that lead solder is no longer used in the manufacture and packaging of canned food for infants. Older children tend however to eat the same food as the adult members of the family and it is important to ensure that permitted levels are kept to the lowest possible values. Such action would also minimise pre-natal exposure through the mother. A review of metals in canned food is currently being undertaken by an independent advisory group, the Food Additives and Contaminants Committee, and we would welcome any proposals for further reductions in the lead content of food.

Lead in Tap Water

189 Results from the Department of Environment survey show that, for some 60 to 70% of the population, drinking water makes no appreciable

contribution to the total intake of lead. With some waters, notably those which are soft and acidic, the levels of lead in water are increased when lead plumbing is used; in a few localities a high intake of lead is attributable to this source. The use of such contaminated water for the preparation of infant milk feeds is of particular concern. The lead content of food can also be increased if such water is used for cooking and food preparation. A national programme is under way with the aim of reducing substantially the levels of lead in affected tap water, primarily by the chemical treatment of plumbo-solvent waters. An upper limit has been proposed for lead in tap water of 100 μg/l as an average in any household, even in the worst affected areas. We were concerned to learn that it is not at present certain that chemical treatment will always be sufficiently effective, particularly with some plumbo-solvent hard waters, and that where lead lined tanks are fitted it will be ineffective. Pipe replacement would not be practicable on a wide scale but it will have to be considered where there is no effective alternative; where drinking water is at present drawn through lead lined tanks, these should be replaced, lined or bypassed. Water which has stood in lead pipes for some hours usually has a substantially higher content of lead than that drawn after flushing. Water drawn from the hot tap is also likely to have a relatively high content of lead; because of the effect of heat on soldered joints this can be true even with a non-lead system.

190 We welcome the action which is being taken to reduce the levels of lead in water. Urgent attention should be given to areas where water lead levels are sufficiently high to have a marked effect on blood lead concentrations in the population and measures should be taken to reduce exposure, especially to infants.

Lead in Air

191 For most people in the UK uptake of lead from air is of a low order and generally much less than that from food and water. The long-term average concentrations to which rural and most urban dwellers are exposed are almost certainly less than 0.5 μg/m^3 and for the rest they probably do not exceed 1 μg/m^3. If it is assumed on the basis of results from experimental studies that each μg/m^3 in the air raises the blood lead concentration by about 2 μg/dl, then with blood leads in the typical range of 10 to 20 μg/dl (derived from all sources) the contribution from air lead for such people would be of the order of 10% and possibly a little more if allowance is made for intake of airborne lead via dust. Doubts remain, however, about the form of the relationship between air lead and amounts in the blood. There are some

'hot spots' where long-term average concentrations may be as high as 6 $\mu g/m^3$; continuous exposure to such air lead concentrations may well make air lead the major contribution to uptake for some individuals. We recommend that further monitoring of lead in air should concentrate on identifying local 'hot spots', whether arising from traffic or from industrial sources and that the extent of the increase in blood lead which results from long-term exposure in such circumstances should be investigated.

192 About 90% of airborne lead is derived from petrol; industrial sources may however contribute appreciably to air lead levels in their immediate vicinity. Although there are indications that in some localities contributions from traffic slightly increase blood lead concentrations, the results of recent surveys among adults and children living near busy road junctions and motorways show that blood lead concentrations are within the limits specified by the EEC. The surveys also show that effects from living close to a smelter or in a leadworker's family on the blood lead of children need not be great but the EEC criteria for blood lead in populations were not met in the case of three groups of children due to local factors related to the lead works. It is therefore clear that there need be little risk of increased intake for people living near a lead works but constant care is needed if emissions are to be kept to acceptably low levels and particular attention may have to be given to scrap yards and some small lead-using industries.

193 On the basis of the information available to us we consider that to avoid the possibility of excessive intake of airborne lead annual average concentrations should not exceed the 2 $\mu g/m^3$ limit suggested by the EEC for places where people are exposed continuously for long periods. We return to the role of lead in petrol and in vehicle emissions in paragraphs 208–209.

Adventitious Sources

194 In some sections of the community a wide variety of sources that are not common to the environment as a whole may be encountered, particularly by children, in and around the home. The main adventitious sources of lead are commonly associated with elevated blood lead concentrations and they are the most important and perhaps the only cause of overt clinical lead poisoning in the non-industrially exposed population in the United Kingdom. We believe that the majority of such cases are preventable.

84

195 Risks of exposure depend on personal and social factors as well as on the presence of lead-containing materials; among such factors believed to be important are the age of the child, his nutritional status, how well he is cared for, the socio-economic status of the family and its ethnic group. The habit of pica is of particular importance. Many of these factors are inter-related and it is not always possible to predict which combination of factors may result in a real as opposed to a potential hazard. Thus, some young children in families in low socio-economic groups may be at increased risk by virtue of residence in an old, poorly maintained home and lack of adequate supervision. Indeed we believe that many cases of lead poisoning from adventitious sources reflect social deprivation.

196 The most important risk is that associated with the presence of old lead-based paint and primers on surfaces in and around houses, or other premises and playgrounds to which young children, and especially those with pica, may have access. In Chapter 9 we recommend a series of measures to minimise exposure from this source. In some localities there are excessive amounts of lead in the soil, for example from former mining or industrial operations, which may also result in increased uptake, especially among young children with pica. Guidelines are being developed for the acceptable lead content of soil in gardens, agricultural land, parks and open spaces, and we strongly support such efforts. Results from a number of surveys have also drawn attention to elevated blood lead concentrations among Asian sections of the community and some cases of lead poisoning have been reported. These risks appear to be related, at least in part, to the use of lead-containing cosmetics or medicines which have been privately imported. The importation and use of these products should be discouraged.

197 Details are given in Chapter 5 of a number of other sources of lead which may affect people in the home and it is clear that unexpected sources are discovered from time to time. The sale of lead-containing consumer products is controlled by a range of regulations but we stress the constant vigilance required to reduce exposure to adventitious sources in and around the home. While risks remain, there is a strong need for an educational programme for parents and health workers to increase awareness of these potential hazards.

198 We have not considered directly the risks of exposure of workers in lead-processing industries and scrap yards to elevated levels of lead, since industrial exposure is the concern of the Health and Safety Executive and outside our terms of reference. We have however considered indirect impacts on the community, such as risks of lead dust being dispersed in the home from the contaminated clothing of workers. Studies among occupationally

exposed groups with elevated blood lead concentrations have made a valuable contribution to our understanding of possible effects of lead; workers with blood lead concentrations hitherto considered to be 'acceptable' form a group which merits further study, since recent reports (Haenninen *et al*, 1978, Baker *et al*, 1979) have drawn attention to the possibility of neurological and other adverse effects among workers with blood lead concentrations below 80 μg/dl.

Effects on Children

199 A large proportion of our time has been devoted to the consideration of the effect of lead on the intelligence, behaviour, attainment and performance of children. While it has long been known that lead in certain concentrations is toxic, it is only comparatively recently that the possibility has been raised that relatively low levels of exposure may result in permanent impairment.

200 There are many medical and social conditions which can cause or contribute to a deficit of measured intelligence. In coming to conclusions on research reports we were aware that exposure to lead is often associated with poor environmental circumstances. In general, children with lower than average intelligence come from families living in depressed areas, where the standards of nutrition and schooling are often low. It is thus difficult to distinguish between the effects of lead and of other factors. Carefully controlled studies with appropriate methods of statistical analysis are essential to the assessment of the relative contribution made by these various factors.

201 The problem of measuring the total lead intake received by a child over a long period has not been solved. The concentration of lead in the blood is generally considered to be the most reliable index of recent exposure to lead. At a blood lead concentration of 15 μg/dl the results will be accurate within ±10%, providing that the quality control is meticulous. Tooth lead is increasingly being used as an indicator of long-term exposure but the concentration of lead varies according to the tooth examined and the part analysed. Again accuracy and precision are exceedingly important. Most of the studies we have seen have relied upon a single measurement of the lead concentration in the blood, without making allowance for the intensity, duration and time of exposure. The source of the lead is rarely determined and the physical condition of the child is often not assessed.

202 Difficulties exist in the measurement of intelligence and behaviour. Intelligence test construction, administration, and the interpretation of results all present problems and the measurement of behaviour relies largely on

rating scales which may lack precision and reflect what is observed in only one situation. Unless the examinations are carried out by one person or all the testers are rigorously trained, there can be considerable variation in the results. We have taken particular notice of studies carried out by Needleman and his colleagues which use tooth lead as a measure of exposure as they are by far the most comprehensive so far undertaken. We have a number of reservations about these and other studies using tooth lead (see Chapter 7).

203 Some studies have also attempted to examine the relationship between lead and hyperactivity and lead and poor educational attainment but in our opinion the design of these studies falls far short of the quality needed to demonstrate effects and we conclude that a clear relationship between an increasing lead burden and either of these conditions has not yet been demonstrated.

204 In two ranges of blood lead concentrations we have no doubt about effects. There is no convincing evidence of deleterious effects at blood lead concentrations below about 35 μg/dl. It might be thought that the dentine lead studies provide a *possible* exception to this statement but, as we have pointed out earlier in this report, there are difficulties in their interpretation and it is not possible to translate dentine lead concentrations into blood lead concentrations. We also have no doubt about the neuropsychological consequences of high concentrations of blood lead. Symptoms of lead poisoning and encephalopathy occur with levels in excess of, say, 80 μg/dl. Permanent brain damage may follow encephalopathy, although prompt effective measures to reduce exposure and also blood lead concentration may reduce the risk of permanent sequelae.

205 It is therefore in the range of blood lead concentrations between 35–80 μg/dl that doubt remains. In the published studies it is customary either to compare the difference between two groups of children, the average blood lead levels being higher in one group than in the other, or to consider blood lead concentrations in several broad groups. There are some studies which report that mean blood lead concentrations in this range are associated with deficits in intellectual functioning of the order of 5 points on the IQ scale, while other studies do not show such an effect. In considering the relative weight to be given to apparently conflicting reports, we note that contrary to usual dose-effect principles there appears to be no consistent relationship between the concentration of blood or tooth lead and the degree of reported intellectual impairment. If there were a causally-linked association one would expect to see such a relationship and its absence lends some support to those reports which have noted no deficit in IQ within the

35–80 μg/dl range of blood lead. At present no single blood concentration of lead within this range can be defined above which an individual child is liable to be harmed. Nevertheless, where a child is found to have a blood lead concentration over 35 μg/dl we would recommend that he or she should be carefully followed up to ascertain the source of the lead and to reduce the exposure of the child and of other persons who might be affected.

206 A number of animal studies have suggested that excessive maternal exposure to lead can cause raised foetal blood lead and subsequent learning difficulties among the offspring. The period of maximum brain growth in animals varies with the species and it is very difficult to extrapolate from animal models to human infants. In humans lead is known to pass the placental barrier and foetal blood lead equates closely with maternal blood lead although concentrations are usually a little lower. There is a need for further research into the important subject of pre-natal exposure to lead and its relationship to the subsequent mental and physical development of the child. Studies carried out so far have not been of the standard of those following the exposure to lead in childhood.

General Conclusions

207 We believe that one of the objectives required by our terms of reference has been attained, in that we have been able to assess the role of lead from petrol in relation to the other sources of lead in the environment. The temptation to recommend its urgent removal is great, especially in view of the statement which opens our Report: 'Lead and its compounds are potentially toxic: the element has no known physiological functions . . .'. But the task given to the Working Party was to assess the evidence of effects of lead from all sources and our conclusions must be based on strictly scientific grounds, though our recommendations are tempered by considerations of prudence. The Working Party was absolved from the need to take into account economic factors and the question of conservation of energy in making its assessment and consequent recommendations.

208 We have seen that in the vast majority of the population airborne lead, including that derived from petrol, is usually a minor contributor to the body burden. Normally, food is the major source and we have seen no evidence that this is substantially enhanced by contamination by airborne lead. However, our attention has been drawn not so much to the bulk of the population among whom, according to recent surveys done in the UK in fulfilment of the EEC directive, blood levels meet the reference values, but to

the small proportion which falls into the upper part of the distribution of blood lead concentrations. There is no indication from the surveys that these relatively raised blood concentrations are due to lead from petrol; they would seem more likely to be due to a miscellany of adventitious sources such as lead-containing paint in and around the home, the use of special cosmetics and medicines containing lead, or to tap water in some localities where the water is especially plumbosolvent and lead plumbing is used. We recognise that there are local 'hot spots' where airborne lead concentrations are high and we advise that such places merit urgent attention.

209 After the most careful consideration, the Working Party is unanimous in advising Government and industry to take steps by which emissions of lead into the air, whether from the use of leaded petrol or from other sources, are progressively reduced provided that such action does not lessen the priority which it believes must continue to be given to reducing the opportunities for ingestion of old lead-containing paint and primers and of other adventitious lead which have been seen to cause demonstrable harm, and to the control of the lead content of some tap waters which have been seen to be clearly associated with raised blood lead concentrations. Although we have seen no firm evidence that the contribution made by lead from petrol has caused harm, yet recognising that any additional contribution is undesirable in persons whose body burden may already be high as a result of absorption of lead from other sources, measures should be taken to keep the annual mean concentration of lead in air to less than 2 $\mu g/m^3$ in places where people are liable to be continuously exposed. Such measures could include further reduction in the lead content of petrol, the use of devices to trap some of the lead within the exhaust system, improvements in traffic flow through traffic management schemes, and the re-location of any industrial operations that create local problems.

210 We have not been able to come to clear conclusions concerning the effects of small amounts of lead on the intelligence, behaviour and performance of children. There are some studies which have failed to demonstrate any effects, and there are others which have yielded positive results, but many of the studies which we have scrutinised do not provide evidence from which valid conclusions can be drawn. We are agreed that adverse effects in children who have, for one reason or another, absorbed undue amounts of lead cannot be discounted. We have made recommendations about increased monitoring, general vigilance, and the development of educational programmes aimed at the identification and increasing awareness of unusual risks from any environmental source; we would add a strong plea for the

9 Recommendations

Recommendations for Action

211 Although these points have not been given any relative weighting the first three listed are those where there is clear evidence that individual exposure to lead in certain circumstances could be high, with potential risk to health. Urgent attention should be directed to these matters. Recommendations 4, 5 and 6 are no less important but the value in further reduction of lead in food and air lies in the need to reduce the cumulative effect from a multiplicity of sources.

(1) There should be a programme for the detection of lead in paint coatings accessible to young children in areas where a high incidence of old lead paint surfaces may be suspected, such as old inner city residential areas. The lead content of all paint available for retail sale, including paint intended for the exterior surfaces of houses and for institutions, schools and play areas should be as low as is technically feasible. Any paint intended for industrial use which contains lead should be labelled to indicate its lead content and its unsuitability for use in and around the home; all possible steps should be taken to discourage the improper use of such paint (paragraphs 69–75).*

(2) The strongest possible support should be given to local authorities and water undertakings in the programme to reduce levels of lead in tap water in affected areas. The reduction should generally be to the maximum extent possible by reasonable means. Priority should be given to effective action in areas where individual exposures to lead from water are markedly high. Pipe replacement, or other adjustments to plumbing, must be considered where there is no effective alternative; in particular, lead lined tanks should be replaced, lined or bypassed. The possibility of making grants available to assist in these circumstances may need to be considered. While special problems still exist in some areas, it should generally be recommended that people in affected households should avoid drawing the first run-off for drinking or

---

*refers to relevant discussion in main text.

food preparation after cold water has stood in the pipes for a few hours or more. Water from hot taps should not be used for these purposes, especially not for preparing infants' feeds. Special attention should be given to affected households where there are babies or expectant mothers and it may even be necessary to make changes to plumbing in an individual dwelling or to supply safe bottled water (Chapter 3).

(3) The private importation and use of lead containing cosmetics should be discouraged and potential users of these products made aware of the hazards which they may present. Hair care preparations which contain lead should state this on the label, together with a warning against misuse (paragraphs 79-85).

(4) Action to eliminate lead contamination of manufactured foods is endorsed, and it is recommended that permitted levels in all foodstuffs be kept as low as practicable (paragraphs 23-30).

(5) Emissions of lead to the air from traffic and other sources should be progressively reduced, subject to an appraisal of any other possible effects on health of altering the constituents of petrol (paragraphs 56-61).

(6) Measures should be taken to keep the annual mean concentration of lead in air to less than 2 μg/m^3 in places where people are liable to be continuously exposed for long periods. These measures may include the reduction of emissions, the relocation of industry or housing, or traffic management schemes (paragraphs 106-107, 193).

(7) There should be maximum vigilance to identify toys for sale which are coated with paint containing lead in excess of the quantity allowed in current regulations (paragraph 75).

(8) Encouragement should be given towards the current development of guidelines for acceptable concentrations of lead in soil in gardens, agricultural land, parks and open spaces (paragraph 77).

(9) The public should be made aware of the potential hazards of imperfectly glazed ceramic ware and of old lead pewter (paragraph 78).

(10) Steps should be taken to give parents and health workers a better understanding of known lead hazards, including the dangers of pica (paragraphs 79, 81, 82, 86-89).

(11) Adequate training, equipment and facilities should be ensured for Medical Officers of Environmental Health and Environmental Health Officers or others responsible for the investigation of domestic lead hazards.

(12) Consideration should be given to the need for co-ordination through a central unit of activity on lead in the fields of environmental monitoring and clinical investigation.

Recommendations for Further Research and Monitoring

(13) The detailed identification of areas with high levels of lead in tap water should be pursued vigorously and technical research to allow intake to be more accurately estimated from water lead measurements should be supported.

(14) Further monitoring of lead in air and dust should concentrate especially on identifying places where people are liable to spend long periods in the presence of high concentrations. Attention should be directed not only to residential areas close to traffic, but also to areas close to industrial sources, including small (and often poorly controlled) sources such as scrap yards.

(15) Surveys to monitor blood lead in the general population should continue, especially in areas with relatively high exposures to lead in water, air and dust.

(16) In the event of any major change in exposures to lead, monitoring programmes for both environmental lead and blood lead should be designed to allow trends to be followed over a number of years.

(17) Since in some cases blood lead determination based on capillary samples can be unreliable, it is recommended that in general venous samples should be used in both clinical and survey work.

(18) Individuals and particularly children, whose blood lead concentrations are found to be over 35 μg/dl should be followed up, in order to identify the source of the lead exposure, and to take appropriate action.

(19) Further research projects should be conducted to investigate relationships between exposure to lead and intelligence, educational attainment and behaviour in children. These may require the development of new testing procedures for studying behavioural aspects. Attention will also need to be given to methods of determining exposure to lead at the relevant time. In this connection, further investigations on the value of analyses on teeth and other tissues may be needed.

(20) Where substantial reductions in exposure are achieved, the effect in terms of changes in psychological functioning as well as in terms of changes in body lead should be studied.

(21) To gain further information on possible effects of moderately elevated levels of lead in adults, more studies among occupationally exposed populations with blood lead levels below 80 μg/dl should be encouraged.

(22) To supplement information obtained from experimental work on the relationship between lead in the environment and blood lead, additional studies, including further work on the alpha factor (α) and on the extent to which airborne lead contributes to blood lead via food, are required.

Membership of the DHSS Working Party on Lead

Chairman

Professor P J Lawther CBE, MB, BS, DSc, FRCP

Professor of Environmental and Preventive Medicine
St Bartholomew's Hospital Medical College
University of London

Members

Dr D Barltrop MD, BSc, FRCP, DCH

Director
Department of Child Health
Westminster Medical School
University of London

Dr R N Chamberlain MB, ChB, FFCM, DCH

Senior Epidemiologist
Central Public Health Laboratory
London

Professor B E Clayton MD, Ph D, FRCP, FRC Path

Professor of Chemical Pathology and Human Metabolism
University of Southampton

Professor W W Holland MD, B Sc, MRCGP, FRCP, FFCM

Professor of Clinical Epidemiology and Social Medicine
St Thomas' Hospital Medical School
University of London

Dr R G Lansdown MA, Ph D

Principal Psychologist
Department of Psychological Medicine
Hospital for Sick Children
London

Dr B Moore MD, B Sc, FRC Path	Honorary Research Fellow Department of Mathematical Statistics and Operational Research University of Exeter
Professor T E Oppe MB, BS, FRCP, DCH	Professor of Paediatrics St Mary's Hospital Medical School University of London
Professor M Rutter MD, FRCP, FRC Psych, DPM	Professor of Child Psychiatry Institute of Psychiatry University of London
Dr H A Waldron MD, Ph D, MRCP, MFOM	Senior Lecturer in Occupational Medicine London School of Hygiene and Tropical Medicine University of London
Mr R E Waller B Sc	Member of MRC Scientific Staff St. Bartholomew's Hospital Medical College University of London
Dr W Yule MA, Dip Psych, Ph D	Senior Lecturer in Psychology Institute of Psychiatry University of London

Secretaries

Dr M F Cuthbert MB, BS, Ph D (Medical Secretary)	Department of Health and Social Security
Mr B G Wrigley (Administrative Secretary)	Department of Health and Social Security

Representatives of the following Government Departments and organisations were in attendance: The Department of the Environment; the Ministry of Agriculture, Fisheries and Food; the Department of Health and Social Security; the Medical Research Council; the Scottish Home and Health Department; the Welsh Office.

EEC Blood Lead Survey

Results from the 1979 UK Campaign

1 The UK campaign was announced in the House of Commons on 22 February 1979. It fulfils the EEC directive 77/312/EEC (Official Journal L105/10,28 April 1977) on the biological screening of the population for lead which calls for two campaigns co-ordinated across the Community and separated by two years. The UK campaign is made up of autonomous surveys carried out by local medical and environmental health authorities on different groups of people. Their work is co-ordinated by the Department of the Environment assisted by other Government Departments. Originally, 42 groups of people in various towns were to take part. During the campaign this was reduced to 39: the results for 2 groups in Bristol were not compatible with the others and the survey of lead workers' children in Dartford comprised only 3 donors, not enough for a statistically valid sample. Results for 2 groups, mothers and their new born babies in Glasgow, will not be available until Spring 1980. The tables reproduced in this Appendix cover the following groups of people:—

Adults in major urban areas	*Persons specifically exposed to lead*
Inner Birmingham (Handsworth)	Beverley—Children of lead workers
Inner Birmingham (Sparkbrook)	
Outer Birmingham (Sutton Coldfield)	Chester—Children of lead workers
	Chester—Children near lead works
Glasgow	
	Dartford—Children near battery works
Inner Leeds	Ellesmere Port—Children of lead workers
Outer Leeds	Ellesmere Port—Children near organic lead works

Inner Liverpool	Gravesham—Children of lead workers
Outer Liverpool	Gravesham—Children near lead works
Inner London (LB Islington)	
Inner London (LB Lambeth)	
Outer London	Leeds (Tingley)—Children near motorway
(LB Kingston upon	Leeds (Thorpe)—Children of lead workers
Thames)	Leeds (Thorpe)—Children near lead works
Outer London	
(LB Waltham Forest)	
Inner Manchester	LB Brent—Adults near North Circular Road
Outer Manchester	LB Greenwich—Children of lead workers
	LB Greenwich—Children near lead works
Inner Sheffield	LB Hillingdon—Adults near M4
Outer Sheffield	LB Hillingdon—Children near M4
	LB Tower Hamlets—Children near main road
	Market Harborough—Children of lead workers
	Market Harborough—Children near battery works
	Newport (Gwent)—Children of lead workers
	Newport (Gwent)—Children near battery works

2 The groups of people studied in the UK fall under three headings prescribed by the Directive:—

Indent 1. randomly selected adults in major urban areas;

Indent 2. persons exposed to significant sources of lead pollution; (comprising, in the UK, children of lead workers, children living near lead-using works, people living near main roads, certain mothers in Glasgow); and

Indent 3. persons at risk special (in the UK, children born to the mothers in Glasgow in Indent 2).

All surveys exclude people exposed to lead in their work.

3 The Directive defines 'reference' levels expressed in microgrammes of lead per 100 millilitres of blood ($\mu g/100ml$) to be applied to each group of people in assessing the results of the survey:—

a maximum of 20 $\mu g/100ml$ for 50% of the group

a maximum of 30 $\mu g/100ml$ for 90% of the group

a maximum of 35 $\mu g/100ml$ for 98% of the group

If the levels are exceeded, the EEC Commission must be told and measures taken to trace and reduce the source(s) of exposure. Any individual whose blood lead exceeds 35 μg/100ml must be told and the environmental circumstances must be investigated. The tables reproduced in this appendix apply the reference levels to the groups reported: the right-hand column in each table gives the percentages of the group of people below each reference level.

4 The Department of the Environment prepared the following notes to accompany the results of the UK surveys:–

Notes on the EEC Blood Lead Results

i. Anybody who was medically followed for occupational exposure to lead should not have been included in the surveys. In a few cases blood samples were taken from people who were medically followed but these blood lead values are not included in the tables.

ii. Repeat blood samples were obtained wherever possible if the first sample was technically unsuitable for analysis or if there was a high blood lead level – generally over 30 μg/100 ml for children and over 35 μg/100 ml for adults. In the surveys where intravenous sampling was practised, the tables reported results for the first analysable specimens obtained. In surveys using a capillary sampling method, the results reported are generally for the first analysable specimens but if repeat (venous) specimens had been taken, their values are reported. The adult surveys all used intravenous sampling, but the children's surveys reported here used both the capillary and intravenous methods; a note on each table indicates the method(s) used.

iii. The tables report the results of analyses by laboratories that had to meet stringent national and international quality control criteria. Throughout the UK campaign strict measures were applied to the participating laboratories of the NHS Supra-Regional Assay Service and an associated laboratory in Scotland to ensure consistency and accuracy of results. If a laboratory's performance fell outside the control limits, its work was repeated by a laboratory within the limits. The tables report only the values determined by the second laboratory.

EEC Blood Lead Survey 1979

Indent 1: Inner Birmingham – Handsworth

Blood lead µg/100ml	Males			Females			Persons		
	No	%	Cum %	No	%	Cum %	No	%	Cum %
Less than or equal to 20	42	76	76	40	91	91	82	83	83
21–30	11	20	96	4	9	100	15	15	98
31–35	—	—	96	—	—	—	—	—	98
Over 35	2	4	100	—	—	—	2	2	100
Total	**55**	**100**	**100**	**44**	**100**	**100**	**99**	**100**	**100**

Notes:

1 This survey meets the reference levels.

2 Blood samples were taken by venepuncture.

EEC Blood Lead Survey 1979

Indent 1: Inner Birmingham – Sparkbrook

Blood lead µg/100ml	Males			Females			Persons		
	No	%	Cum %	No	%	Cum %	No	%	Cum %
Less than or equal to 20	35	76	76	49	96	96	84	87	87
21–30	11	24	100	2	4	100	13	13	100
31–35	—	—	—	—	—	—	—	—	—
Over 35	—	—	—	—	—	—	—	—	—
Total	**46**	**100**	**100**	**51**	**100**	**100**	**97[2]**	**100**	**100**

Notes:

1 This survey meets the reference levels.

2 A further 2 results were received but were excluded from the table since the respondents were medically followed for occupational exposure to lead. Their blood lead levels were 57 µg/100ml and 13 µg/100ml.

3 Blood samples were taken by venepuncture.

EEC Blood Lead Survey 1979
Indent 1: Outer Birmingham

Blood lead µg/100ml	Males			Females			Persons		
	No	%	Cum %	No	%	Cum %	No	%	Cum %
Less than or equal to 20	43	93	93	53	98	98	96	96	96
21–30	3	7	100	1	2	100	4	4	100
31–35	—	—	—	—	—	—	—	—	—
Over 35	—	—	—	—	—	—	—	—	—
Total	**46**	**100**	**100**	**54**	**100**	**100**	**100**	**100**	**100**

Notes:

1 This survey meets the reference levels.

2 Blood samples were taken by venepuncture.

EEC Blood Lead Survey 1979
Indent 1: Glasgow

Blood lead µg/100ml	Males			Females			Persons		
	No	%	Cum %	No	%	Cum %	No	%	Cum %
Less than or equal to 20	55	56	56	79	81	81	134	68	68
21–30	32	33	89	16	16	97	48	24	92
31–35	5	5	94	2	2	99	7	4	96
Over 35	6	6	100	1	1	100	7	4	100
Total	**98**	**100**	**100**	**98**	**100**	**100**	**196**	**100**	**100**

Notes:

1 Since more than 2% of the sample had blood lead levels above 35 µg/100ml, this survey does not meet the reference levels.

2 Blood samples were taken by venepuncture.

3 A further 2 forms were received but were excluded from the table since the respondents were medically followed for occupational exposure to lead. Their blood lead levels were 28 µg/100ml and 38 µg/100ml.

EEC Blood Lead Survey 1979

Indent 1: Inner Leeds

Blood lead µg/100ml	Males			Females			Persons		
	No	%	Cum %	No	%	Cum %	No	%	Cum %
Less than or equal to 20	39	71	71	39	87	87	79[2]	78	78
21–30	14	25	96	5	11	98	19	19	97
31–35	—	—	96	1	2	100	1	1	98
Over 35	2	4	100	—	—	—	2	2	100
Total	**55**	**100**	**100**	**45**	**100**	**100**	**101**	**100**	**100**

Notes:

1 This survey meets the reference levels.

2 Includes one person whose sex was not reported on the questionnaire.

3 Blood samples were taken by venepuncture.

EEC Blood Lead Survey 1979

Indent 1: Outer Leeds

Blood lead µg/100ml	Males			Females			Persons		
	No	%	Cum %	No	%	Cum %	No	%	Cum %
Less than or equal to 20	36	80	80	54	96	96	90	89	89
21–30	9	20	100	2	4	100	11	11	100
31–35	—	—	—	—	—	—	—	—	—
Over 35	—	—	—	—	—	—	—	—	—
Total	**45**	**100**	**100**	**56**	**100**	**100**	**101**	**100**	**100**

Notes:

1 This survey meets the reference levels.

2 Blood samples were taken by venepuncture.

EEC Blood Lead Survey 1979
Indent 1: Inner Liverpool

Blood lead µg/100ml	Males			Females			Persons		
	No	%	Cum %	No	%	Cum %	No	%	Cum %
Less than or equal to 20	34	79	79	52	91	91	86	86	86
21–30	8	19	98	4	7	98	12	12	98
31–35	1	2	100	1	2	100	2	2	100
Over 35	—	—	—	—	—	—	—	—	—
Total	**43**	**100**	**100**	**57**	**100**	**100**	**100**	**100**	**100**

Notes:

1 This survey meets the reference levels.

2 Blood samples were taken by venepuncture.

EEC Blood Lead Survey 1979
Indent 1: Outer Liverpool

Blood lead µg/100ml	Males			Females			Persons		
	No	%	Cum %	No	%	Cum %	No	%	Cum %
Less than or equal to 20	27	73	73	59	94	94	86	86	86
21–30	7	19	92	4	6	100	11	11	97
31–35	1	3	95	—	—	—	1	1	98
Over 35	2	5	100	—	—	—	2	2	100
Total	**37**	**100**	**100**	**63**	**100**	**100**	**100**	**100**	**100**

Notes:

1 This survey meets the reference levels.

2 Blood samples were taken by venepuncture.

EEC Blood Lead Survey 1979
Indent 1: Islington [Inner London]

Blood lead μg/100ml	Males			Females			Persons		
	No	%	Cum. %	No	%	Cum. %	No	%	Cum. %
Less than or equal to 20	35	90	90	47	98	98	82	94	94
21–30	2	5	95	1	2	100	3	3	98
31–35	2	5	100	—	—	—	2	2	100
Over 35	—	—	—	—	—	—	—	—	—
Total	**39**	**100**	**100**	**48**	**100**	**100**	**87**	**100**	**100**

Notes:

1 This survey meets the reference levels.

2 Percentages have been rounded independently and therefore may not sum to totals shown.

3 Blood samples were taken by venepuncture.

EEC Blood Lead Survey 1979
Indent 1: Lambeth [Inner London]

Blood lead μg/100ml	Males			Females			Persons		
	No	%	Cum. %	No	%	Cum. %	No	%	Cum. %
Less than or equal to 20	86	91	91	103	98	98	189	95	95
21–30	8	8	99	2	2	100	10	5	100
31–35	—	—	99	—	—	—	—	—	100
Over 35	1	1	100	—	—	—	1	1	100
Total	**95**	**100**	**100**	**105**	**100**	**100**	**200**	**100**	**100**

Notes:

1 This survey meets the reference levels.

2 Percentages have been rounded independently and therefore may not sum to 100.

3 Blood samples were taken by venepuncture.

EEC Blood Lead Survey 1979
Indent 1: Kingston upon Thames [Outer London]

Blood lead µg/100ml	Males			Females			Persons		
	No	%	Cum. %	No	%	Cum. %	No	%	Cum. %
Less than or equal to 20	112	92	92	36	100	100	148	94	94
21–30	10	8	100	—	—	—	10	6	100
31–35	—	—	—	—	—	—	—	—	—
Over 35	—	—	—	—	—	—	—	—	—
Total	**122**	**100**	**100**	**36**	**100**	**100**	**158**	**100**	**100**

Notes:

1 This survey meets the reference levels.

2 A further 10 samples were not sufficient for analysis.

3 Blood samples were taken by venepuncture.

EEC Blood Lead Survey 1979
Indent 1: Waltham Forest [Outer London]

Blood lead µg/100ml	Males			Females			Persons		
	No	%	Cum. %	No	%	Cum. %	No	%	Cum. %
Less than or equal to 20	89	94	94	102	100	100	191	97	97
21–30	6	6	100	—	—	—	6	3	100
31–35	—	—	—	—	—	—	—	—	—
Over 35	—	—	—	—	—	—	—	—	—
Total	**95**	**100**	**100**	**102**	**100**	**100**	**197**	**100**	**100**

Notes:

1 This survey meets the reference levels.

2 Blood samples were taken by venepuncture.

EEC Blood Lead Survey 1979
Indent 1: Inner Manchester

Blood lead µg/100ml	Males			Females			Persons		
	No	%	Cum %	No	%	Cum %	No	%	Cum %
Less than or equal to 20	26	57	57	45	83	83	71	71	71
21–30	17	37	93	9	17	100	26	26	97
31–35	1	2	96	—	—	—	1	1	98
Over 35	2	4	100	—	—	—	2	2	100
Total	**46**	**100**	**100**	**54**	**100**	**100**	**100**	**100**	**100**

Notes:

1 This survey meets the reference levels.

2 Blood samples were taken by venepuncture.

EEC Blood Lead Survey 1979
Indent 1: Outer Manchester

Blood lead µg/100ml	Males			Females			Persons		
	No	%	Cum %	No	%	Cum %	No	%	Cum %
Less than or equal to 20	36	72	72	39	76	76	75	74	74
21–30	11	22	94	11	22	98	22	22	96
31–35	3	6	100	1	2	100	4	4	100
Over 35	—	—	—	—	—	—	—	—	—
Total	**50**	**100**	**100**	**51**	**100**	**100**	**101**	**100**	**100**

Notes:

1 This survey meets the reference levels.

2 Percentages have been rounded independently and therefore may not sum to totals shown.

3 Blood samples were taken by venepuncture.

EEC Blood Lead Survey–1979
Indent 1: Inner Sheffield

Blood lead µg/100ml	Males			Females			Persons		
	No	%	Cum %	No	%	Cum %	No	%	Cum %
Less than or equal to 20	44	85	85	47	98	98	91	91	91
21–30	8	15	100	1	2	100	9	9	100
31–35	—	—	—	—	—	—	—	—	—
Over 35	—	—	—	—	—	—	—	—	—
Total	**52**	**100**	**100**	**48**	**100**	**100**	**100**	**100**	**100**

Notes:

1 This survey meets the reference levels.

2 Blood samples were taken by venepuncture.

EEC Blood Lead Survey 1979
Indent 1: Outer Sheffield

Blood lead µg/100ml	Males			Females			Persons		
	No	%	Cum %	No	%	Cum %	No	%	Cum %
Less than or equal to 20	43	91	91	51	98	98	95[2]	95	95
21–30	4	9	100	1	2	100	5	5	100
31–35	—	—	—	—	—	—	—	—	—
Over 35	—	—	—	—	—	—	—	—	—
Total	**47**	**100**	**100**	**52**	**100**	**100**	**100**	**100**	**100**

Notes:

1 This survey meets the reference levels.

2 Includes one person whose sex was not reported on the questionnaire.

3 Blood samples were taken by venepuncture.

EEC Blood Lead Survey 1979
Indent 2: Beverley – Lead Workers' Children

Blood lead µg/100ml	Males			Females			Persons		
	No	%	Cum %	No	%	Cum %	No	%	Cum %
Less than or equal to 20	55	80	80	57	88	88	112	84	84
21–30	14	20	100	8	12	100	22	16	100
31–35	—	—	—	—	—	—	—	—	—
Over 35	—	—	—	—	—	—	—	—	—
Total	69	100	100	65	100	100	134	100	100

Notes:

1 This survey meets the reference levels.

2 Blood samples were taken by the capillary method.

EEC Blood Lead Survey 1979
Indent 2: Chester–Children of Leadworkers

Blood lead µg/100ml	Males			Females			Persons		
	No	%	Cum %	No	%	Cum %	No	%	Cum %
Less than or equal to 20	24	62	62	22	55	55	46	58	58
21–30	14	36	97	11	28	83	26[2]	33	90
31–35	1	3	100	2	5	88	3	4	94
Over 35	—	—	—	5	13	100	5	6	100
Total	39	100	100	40	100	100	80	100	100

Notes:

1 Since more than 2% of the sample had blood lead levels above 35 µg/100ml, this survey does not meet the reference levels.

2 Includes one child whose sex was not recorded on the questionnaire.

3 Percentages have been rounded independently and therefore may not sum to totals shown.

4 The vast majority of the blood samples were taken by venepuncture. A small number of samples at the beginning of the survey were taken by the capillary method.

EEC Blood Lead Survey 1979

Indent 2: Chester – Children living near Leadworks

Blood lead µg/100ml	Males			Females			Persons		
	No	%	Cum %	No	%	Cum %	No	%	Cum %
Less than or equal to 20	30	51	51	24	60	60	54	55	55
21–30	22	37	88	15	38	98	37	37	92
31–35	1	2	90	—	—	98	1	1	93
Over 35	6	10	100	1	3	100	7	7	100
Total	**59**	**100**	**100**	**40**	**100**	**100**	**99**	**100**	**100**

Notes.

1 Since more than 2% of the sample had blood lead levels above 35 µg/100ml, this survey does not meet the reference levels.

2 Percentages have been rounded independently and therefore may not sum to totals shown.

3 The vast majority of the samples were taken by venepuncture.

4 A further 58 samples were received from children who attended schools near the leadworks, but who lived more than 1000 metres from the works. These results were excluded from the table and were distributed as follows:-

Blood lead µg/100ml	Males		Females		Persons	
	No	%	No	%	No	%
Less than 20	21	81	27	84	48	83
21–30	5	19	5	16	10	17
Over 30	—	—	—	—	—	—
Total	**26**	**100**	**32**	**100**	**58**	**100**

EEC Blood Lead Survey 1979

Indent 2: Dartford – Children living near Battery Works

Blood lead µg/100ml	Males			Females			Persons		
	No	%	Cum %	No	%	Cum %	No	%	Cum %
Less than or equal to 20	29	85	85	18	78	78	47	82	82
21–30	4	12	97	4	17	96	8	14	96
31–35	1	3	100	1	4	100	2	4	100
Over 35	—	—	—	—	—	—	—	—	—
Total	34	100	100	23	100	100	57	100	100

Notes:

1 This survey meets the reference levels.

2 A further 3 results were excluded from the table since the respondents were also children of battery workers. Their blood lead levels were 27 µg/100ml, 29 µg/100ml and 33 µg/100ml.

3 Blood samples were taken by venepuncture.

4 Percentages have been rounded independently and therefore may not sum to totals shown.

EEC Blood Lead Survey 1979

Indent 2: Ellesmere Port–Children of Leadworkers

Blood lead µg/100ml	Males			Females			Persons		
	No	%	Cum %	No	%	Cum %	No	%	Cum %
Less than or equal to 20	18	90	90	13	100	100	31	94	94
21–30	2	10	100	—	—	—	2	6	100
31–35	—	—	—	—	—	—	—	—	—
Over 35	—	—	—	—	—	—	—	—	—
Total	20	100	100	13	100	100	33	100	100

Notes:

1 This survey meets the reference levels.

2 Blood samples were taken by venepuncture.

EEC Blood Lead Survey 1979

Indent 2: Ellesmere Port – Children living near Lead Works

Blood lead µg/100ml	Males			Females			Persons		
	No	%	Cum %	No	%	Cum %	No	%	Cum %
Less than or equal to 20	29	94	94	28	80	80	57	86	86
21–30	2	6	100	7	20	100	9	14	100
31–35	—	—	—	—	—	—	—	—	—
Over 35	—	—	—	—	—	—	—	—	—
Total	**31**	**100**	**100**	**35**	**100**	**100**	**66**	**100**	**100**

Notes:
1 This survey meets the reference levels.
2 Blood samples were taken by venepuncture.

EEC Blood Lead Survey 1979

Indent 2: Gravesham – Children of Leadworkers

Blood lead µg/100ml	Males			Females			Persons		
	No	%	Cum %	No	%	Cum %	No	%	Cum %
Less than or equal to 20	52	57	57	51	57	57	104[2]	57	57
21–30	37	40	97	35	39	96	73[3]	40	96
31–35	2	2	99	3	3	99	5	3	99
Over 35	1	1	100	1	1	100	2	1	100
Total	**92**	**100**	**100**	**90**	**100**	**100**	**184**	**100**	**100**

Notes:
1 This survey meets the references levels.
2,3 Each of these rows includes a child whose sex was not reported on the questionnaire.
4 Percentages have been rounded independently and therefore may not sum to 100.
5 Blood samples were taken by the capillary method.

111

EEC Blood Lead Survey 1979

Indent 2: Gravesham – Children living near Leadworks

Blood lead µg/100ml	Males			Females			Persons		
	No	%	Cum %	No	%	Cum %	No	%	Cum %
Less than or equal to 20	26	81	81	27	93	93	53	87	87
21–30	6	19	100	2	7	100	8	13	100
31–35	—	—	—	—	—	—	—	—	—
Over 35	—	—	—	—	—	—	—	—	—
Total	32	100	100	29	100	100	61	100	100

Notes:

1 This survey meets the reference levels.

2 A further 36 control samples were received but were excluded from the table since the respondents lived more than 1000 metres from the lead works. The blood lead levels of these respondents were distributed as follows:

Blood lead µg/100ml	Males		Females		Persons	
	No	%	No	%	No	%
Less than or equal to 20	22	100	14	100	36	100
Over 20	—	—	—	—	—	—
Total	22	100	14	100	36	100

3 Blood samples were taken by the capillary method.

EEC Blood Lead Survey 1979

Indent 2: Tingley – Children living near Motorway Interchange

Blood lead µg/100ml	Males			Females			Persons		
	No	%	Cum. %	No	%	Cum. %	No	%	Cum. %
Less than or equal to 20	135	100	100	138	98	98	274[2]	99	99
21–30	—	—	—	3	2	100	3	1	100
31–35	—	—	—	—	—	—	—	—	—
Over 35	—	—	—	—	—	—	—	—	—
Total	135	100	100	141	100	100	277	100	100

Notes:

1 This survey meets the reference levels.

2 Includes one child whose sex was not reported on the questionnaire.

3 Blood samples were taken by venepuncture.

EEC Blood Lead Survey 1979

Indent 2: Thorpe, Leeds – Children of Leadworkers

Blood lead µg/100ml	Males			Females			Persons		
	No	%	Cum. %	No	%	Cum. %	No	%	Cum. %
Less than or equal to 20	21	68	68	29	83	83	50	76	76
21–30	8	26	94	5	14	97	13	20	95
31–35	1	3	97	—	—	97	1	2	97
Over 35	1	3	100	1	3	100	2	3	100
Total	31	100	100	35	100	100	66	100	100

Notes:

1 Since more than 2% of the sample had blood lead levels above 35µg/100ml this survey does not meet the reference levels.

2 Percentages have been rounded independently and therefore may not sum to totals shown.

3 Blood samples were taken by venepuncture.

EEC Blood Lead Survey 1979
Indent 2: Thorpe, Leeds – Children living near Leadworks

Blood lead µg/100ml	Males			Females			Persons		
	No	%	Cum. %	No	%	Cum. %	No	%	Cum. %
Less than or equal to 20	79	90	90	88	97	97	170[2]	93	93
21–30	9	10	100	3	3	100	13[3]	7	100
31–35	—	—	—	—	—	—	—	—	—
Over 35	—	—	—	—	—	—	—	—	—
Total	**88**	**100**	**100**	**91**	**100**	**100**	**183**	**100**	**100**

Notes:

1 This survey meets the reference levels.

2 Includes 3 children whose sex was not reported on the questionnaire.

3 Includes 1 child whose sex was not reported on the questionnaire.

4 Percentages have been rounded independently and therefore may not sum to totals shown.

5 Blood samples were taken by venepuncture.

EEC Blood Lead Survey 1979
Indent 2: Brent – Adults living near North Circular Road

Blood lead µg/100ml	Males			Females			Persons		
	No	%	Cum. %	No	%	Cum. %	No	%	Cum. %
Less than or equal to 20	90	91	91	94	100	100	184	95	95
21–30	8	8	99	—	—	—	8	4	99
31–35	—	—	99	—	—	—	—	—	99
Over 35	1	1	100	—	—	—	1	1	100
Total	**99**	**100**	**100**	**94**	**100**	**100**	**193[2]**	**100**	**100**

Notes:

1 This survey meets the reference levels.

2 A further 3 blood samples were not sufficient for analysis.

3 Blood samples were taken by venepuncture.

EEC Blood Lead Survey 1979

Indent 2: Greenwich – Children of Leadworkers

Blood lead µg/100ml	Males			Females			Persons		
	No	%	Cum %	No	%	Cum %	No	%	Cum %
Less than or equal to 20	37	86	86	40	91	91	77	89	89
21–30	6	14	100	4	9	100	10	11	100
31–35	—	—	—	—	—	—	—	—	—
Over 35	—	—	—	—	—	—	—	—	—
Total	**43**	**100**	**100**	**44**	**100**	**100**	**87**	**100**	**100**

Notes:

1 This survey meets the reference levels.

2 Blood samples were taken by venepuncture.

EEC Blood Lead Survey 1979

Indent 2: Greenwich – Children living near Leadworks

Blood lead µg/100ml	Males			Females			Persons		
	No	%	Cum %	No	%	Cum %	No	%	Cum %
Less than or equal to 20	170	89	89	192	93	93	366[3]	92	92
21–30	20	11	100	12	6	99	32	8	99
31–35	—	—	—	1 }	1 }	100	1 }	1 }	100
Over 35	—	—	—	1 }			1 }		
Total	**190**	**100**	**100**	**206**	**100**	**100**	**400**	**100**	**100**

Notes:

1 This survey meets the reference levels.

2 Percentages have been rounded independenty and therefore may not sum to totals shown.

3 Includes 4 children whose sex was not reported on the questionnaires.

4 Blood samples were taken by venepuncture.

EEC Blood Lead Survey 1979

Indent 2: Hillingdon – Adults living near M.4

Blood lead µg/100ml	Males			Females			Persons		
	No	%	Cum %	No	%	Cum %	No	%	Cum %
Less than or equal to 20	39	75	75	48	92	92	87	84	84
21–30	13	25	100	4	8	100	17	16	100
31–35	—	—	—	—	—	—	—	—	—
Over 35	—	—	—	—	—	—	—	—	—
Total	**52**	**100**	**100**	**52**	**100**	**100**	**104**	**100**	**100**

Notes:

1 This survey meets the reference levels.
2 One further blood sample was insufficient for analysis.
3 Blood samples were taken by the capillary method.

EEC Blood Lead Survey 1979

Indent 2: Hillingdon – Children living near M.4

Blood lead µg/100ml	Males			Females			Persons		
	No	%	Cum %	No	%	Cum %	No	%	Cum %
Less than or equal to 20	28	64	64	32	67	67	60	65	65
21–30	15	34	98	16	33	100	31	34	99
31–35	—	—	98	—	—	—	—	—	99
Over 35	1	2	100	—	—	—	1	1	100
Total	**44**	**100**	**100**	**48**	**100**	**100**	**92**	**100**	**100**

Notes:

1 This survey meets the reference levels.
2 Blood samples were taken by the capillary method.

116

EEC Blood Lead Survey 1979

Indent 2: Tower Hamlets – Children living near Main Road

Blood lead µg/100ml	Males			Females			Persons		
	No	%	Cum %	No	%	Cum %	No	%	Cum %
Less than or equal to 20	75	72	72	52	66	66	127	69	69
21–30	28	27	99	26	33	99	54	30	99
31–35	1	1	100	1	1	100	2	1	100
Over 35	—	—	—	—	—	—	—	—	—
Total	**104**	**100**	**100**	**79**	**100**	**100**	**183**[2]	**100**	**100**

Notes:

1 This survey meets the reference levels.

2 A further 20 blood samples were not sufficient for analysis.

3 Blood samples were taken by the capillary method.

EEC Blood Lead Survey 1979

Indent 2: Market Harborough – Children of Leadworkers

Blood lead µg/100ml	Males			Females			Persons		
	No	%	Cum %	No	%	Cum %	No	%	Cum %
Less than or equal to 20	17	77	77	21	75	75	38	76	76
21–30	5	23	100	6	21	96	11	22	98
31–35	—	—	—	1	4	100	1	2	100
Over 35	—	—	—	—	—	—	—	—	—
Total	**22**	**100**	**100**	**28**	**100**	**100**	**50**[2]	**100**	**100**

Notes:

1 This survey meets the reference levels.

2 A further 3 blood samples were not sufficient for analysis.

3 Blood samples were taken by the capillary method.

EEC Blood Lead Survey 1979
Indent 2: Market Harborough – Children living near Leadworks

Blood lead µg/100ml	Males			Females			Persons		
	No	%	Cum %	No	%	Cum %	No	%	Cum %
Less than or equal to 20	55	76	76	42	76	76	97	76	76
21–30	17	24	100	11	20	96	28	22	98
31–35	—	—	—	1	2	98	1	1	99
Over 35	—	—	—	1	2	100	1	1	100
Total	72	100	100	55	100	100	127[2]	100	100

Notes:

1 This survey meets the reference levels.

2 A further 19 blood samples were not sufficient for analysis.

3 Blood samples were taken by the capillary method.

EEC Blood Lead Survey 1979
Indent 2: Newport – Children of Leadworkers

Blood lead µg/100ml	Males			Females			Persons		
	No	%	Cum %	No	%	Cum %	No	%	Cum %
Less than or equal to 20	19	70	70	13	54	54	32	63	63
21–30	8	30	100	9	38	92	17	33	96
31–35	—	—	—	2	8	100	2	4	100
Over 35	—	—	—	—	—	—	—	—	—
Total	27	100	100	24	100	100	51	100	100

Notes:

1 This survey meets the reference levels.

2 Blood samples were taken by the capillary method.

118

EEC Blood Lead Survey 1979

Indent 2: Newport – Children living near Leadworks

Blood lead µg/100ml	Males			Females			Persons		
	No	%	Cum %	No	%	Cum %	No	%	Cum %
Less than or equal to 20	84	84	84	61	88	88	146[2]	86	86
21–30	16	16	100	7	10	98	23	14	99
31–35	—	—	—	—	—	98	—	—	99
Over 35	—	—	—	1	1	100	1	1	100
Total	**100**	**100**	**100**	**69**	**100**	**100**	**170**	**100**	**100**

Notes:

1 This survey meets the reference levels.

2 Includes one child whose sex was not reported on the questionnaire.

3 Percentages have been rounded independently and therefore may not sum to 100.

4 Blood samples were taken by the capillary method.

Requirements for Cause and Effect Relationships

(BASED ON *A SHORT TEXTBOOK OF MEDICAL STATISTICS* BY AUSTIN BRADFORD HILL, HODDER & STOUGHTON, 1977.)

1 *Strength of the Association*

Consideration of the relative incidence of the condition under study in the populations contrasted. Thus to take a specific example, prospective enquiries into smoking have shown that the death rate from cancer of the lung in cigarette smokers is 9–10 times the rate in non-smokers while the rate in heavy cigarette smokers is 20–30 times as great.

On the other hand, the death rate from coronary thrombosis in smokers appears to be no more than twice, possibly less, the death rate in non-smokers.

2 *Consistency of the Observed Association*

Has it been repeatedly observed by different persons in different places, different circumstances and time? Different results of a different enquiry certainly cannot be held to refute the original evidence. Yet the same results from precisely the same form of enquiry will not invariably greatly strengthen the original evidence. Much weight should be put upon similar results reached in quite different ways, eg in prospective and retrospective enquiries.

3 *Specificity of the Association*

If the association is limited to specific workers and to particular sites and types of disease and there is no association between the work and other modes of dying, then clearly that is a strong argument in favour of causation.

4 *Relationship in time*

5 Biological Gradient or Dose Response Curve

Thus, the fact that the death rate from cancer of the lung has been shown to rise linearly with the number of cigarettes smoked daily adds a very great deal to the simpler evidence that cigarette smokers have a higher death rate than non-smokers.

6 Biological Plausibility

It is helpful if the causation suspected is biologically plausible, though this is a feature that cannot be demanded. What is biologically plausible depends upon the biological knowledge of the day.

7 Coherence of the evidence

The cause and interpretation of an association should not seriously conflict with the general known facts of the natural history and biology of the disease. It should have coherence.

8 The Experiment

Occasionally it is possible to appeal to experimental or semi-experimental evidence. For example, because of an observed association some preventive action is taken. Does it in fact prevent?

9 Reasoning by Analogy

Finally, it would be fair to judge by analogy. With the known effects of the drug Thalidomide and the disease Rubella, we would be ready to accept slighter but similar evidence with another drug or another viral disease in pregnancy.

Clearly, none of these nine viewpoints can bring indisputable evidence for or against the cause and effect hypothesis and equally none can be required as a *sine qua non*. What they can do with greater or less strength, is to help us to answer the fundamental question; is there any other way of explaining the set of facts before us; is there any other answer equally or more likely than cause and effect?

References

ALBERT, R.E., SHORE, R.E., SAYERS, A.J., STREHLOW, C., KNEIP, T.J., PASTERNACK, B.S., FRIEDHOFF, A.J., COVAN, F. and CIMINO, J.A., 1974, Environmental Health Perspectives, 7, 33.

ALEXANDER, F.W., DELVES, H.T. and CLAYTON, B.E., 1973, Commission of the European Communities/United States Environmental Protection Agency: International Symposium on Environmental Health Aspects: of Lead, Amsterdam, 2–6 October, 1972, Luxembourg, p 319.

ALI, A.R., SMALES, O.R.C. and ASLAM, M., 1978, British Medical Journal, 2, 915.

APLING, A.J., CLARK, A.G., ROGERS, F.S.M. and SULLIVAN, E.J., 1979a, Report Nos LR 334–336 (AP), Warren Spring Laboratory, Stevenage, Hertfordshire.

APLING, A.J., ROGERS, F.S.M., SULLIVAN, E.J. and TURNER, A.C., 1979b, Report No LR 338 (AP), Warren Spring Laboratory, Stevenage, Hertfordshire.

ASLAM, M., DAVIS, S.S. and HEALY, M.A., 1979, Public Health (London), 93, 274.

AZAR, A., SNEE, R.D. and HABIBI, K., 1975, Environmental Quality and Safety Supplement, 2, 254.

BAKER, E.L., FOLLAND, D.S., TAYLOR, T.A., FRANK, M., PATERSON, W., LOVEJOY, G., COX, D., HOUSWORTH, J. and LANDRIGAN, P.J., 1977, New England Journal of Medicine, 296, 260.

BAKER, E.L., LANDRIGAN, P.J., BARBOUR, A.G., COX, D.H., FOLLAND, D.S., LIGO, R.N. and THROCKMORTON, J., 1979, British Journal of Industrial Medicine, 36, 314.

BALOH, R., STURM, R., GREEN, B. and GLESER, G., 1975, Archives of Neurology, 32, 326.

BANNISTER, P., 1975, Proceedings of 3rd Unigate Paediatric Workshop: Paediatrics in the Environment, p 35.

BARLTROP, D., 1966, American Journal of Diseases of Children, 112, 116.

BARLTROP, D., 1975, Archives of Industrial Hygiene and Toxicology, 26 (Supplement), 81.

BARLTROP, D., BURMAN, D. and TUCKER, S., 1976, Archives of Diseases in Childhood, 51, 809.

BARLTROP, D. and KHOO, H.E., 1976, Science of the Total Environment, 6, 265.

BARLTROP, D. and KILLALA, N.J.P., 1969, Archives of Diseases in Childhood, 44, 476.

BARLTROP, D. and STREHLOW, C.D., 1978, in Proceedings of the 3rd International Symposium Trace Element Metabolism in Man and Animals (ed Kirchgessner, M.), p 332.

BARLTROP, D., STREHLOW, C.D., THORNTON, I. and WEBB, J.S., 1975, Postgraduate Medical Journal, 51, 801.

BEATTIE, A.D., MOORE, M.R., GOLDBERG, A., FINLAYSON, M.J.W., GRAHAM, J.F., MACKIE, E.M., MAIN, J.C., McLAREN, D.A., MURDOCH R.M. and STEWART, G.T., 1975, Lancet, i, 589.

BERLIN A., AMAVIS, R. and LANGEVIN, M., 1977, in Report of the Meeting of Working Group convened by World Health Organisation Regional Office for Europe, Health Hazards from Drinking Water, 26–30 September, London.

BEVAN, M.G., COLWILL, D.M. and HOGBIN, L.E., 1974, Transport and Road Research Laboratory Report No. 626, Crowthorne, Berkshire.

BICKNELL, J., 1975. Pica. A Childhood symptom, Butterworths, London.

BILLICK, I.H., CURRAN, A.S. and SHIER, D.R., 1979, submitted for publication.

BILLICK, I.H. and GRAY, V.E., 1978. Lead Based Paint Poisoning Research. Review and Evaluation 1971–1977. United States Department of Housing and Urban Development, Washington.

BLAKE, K.C.H., 1976. Environmental Research, 11, 1.

BRADLEY, J.E., POWELL, A.E., NIERMANN, W., McGRADY, K.R. and KAPLAN, E., 1956, Journal of Pediatrics, 49, 1.

BREARLEY, R.L. and FORSYTHE, A.M., 1978, British Medical Journal, 2, 1748.

BULLOCK, J. and LEWIS, W.M., 1968, Atmospheric Environment, 2, 517.

BYERS, R.K. and LORD, E.E., 1943, American Journal of Diseases of Children, 66, 471.

CHAMBERLAIN, A.C., HEARD, M.J., LITTLE, P., NEWTON, D., WELLS, A.C. and WIFFEN, R.D., 1978. Atomic Energy Research Establishment Report R 9198, HMSO.

CHISOLM, J.J. and BARLTROP, D., 1979, Archives of Diseases in Childhood, 54, 249.

CHISOLM, J.J. and HARRISON, H.E., 1956, Pediatrics, 18, 943.

COOPER, M., 1957, Pica, Thomas, Springfield, Illinois.

COSMETICS PRODUCTS REGULATIONS, 1978, Statutory Instrument No. 1354.

COUNCIL OF THE EUROPEAN COMMUNITIES, 1977, Official Journal of the European Communities, L 105, 10.

DAVID, O.J., CLARK, J. and VOELLER, K., 1972, Lancet, ii, 900.

DAVID, O.J., HOFFMAN, S. and KAGEY, B., 1978, in Proceedings of the Symposium on Lead Pollution – Health Effects, Conservation Society, London, p 29.

DAVID, O.J., HOFFMAN, S., McGANN, B., SVERD, J. and CLARK, J., 1976a. Lancet, ii, 1376.

DAVID, O.J., HOFFMAN, S., SVERD, J. and CLARK, J., 1977, Journal of Abnormal Child Psychology, 5, 405.

DAVID, O.J., HOFFMAN, S., SVERD, J., CLARK, J. and VOELLER, K., 1976b, American Journal of Psychiatry, 133, 1155.

De La BURDE, B. and CHOATE, M.S., 1972, Journal of Pediatrics, 81, 1088.

De La BURDE, B. and CHOATE, M.S., 1975, Journal of Pediatrics, 87, 638.

DEPARTMENT OF THE ENVIRONMENT, 1974, Lead in the Environment and its Significance to Man, Pollution Paper No. 2. HMSO, London.

DEPARTMENT OF THE ENVIRONMENT, 1977, Lead in Drinking Water. A Survey in Great Britain, 1975–1976, Pollution Paper No. 12, HMSO, London.

DEPARTMENT OF THE ENVIRONMENT, 1978, Lead Pollution in Birmingham, Pollution Paper No. 14, HMSO, London.

DEPARTMENT OF THE ENVIRONMENT, 1979, Digest of Environmental Pollution Statistics, HMSO, London.

DICKINS, D. and FORD, R.N., 1942, American Sociology Reviews, 7, 59.

FACCHETTI, S., 1979, International Conference on Management and Control of Heavy Metals in the Environment, London, September 1979, CEP Consultants Ltd, Edinburgh, p 95.

FELDMAN, R.G., 1978, New England Journal of Medicine, 298, 1143.

FERNANDES, M.T., 1969, Medical Officer, 122, 88.

FOOD AND AGRICULTURE ORGANISATION/WORLD HEALTH ORGANISATION, 1972, 16th Report of the Joint FAO/WHO Expert Committee on Food Additives, WHO Technical Report Series No 505, Geneva.

GARNYS, V.P., FREEMAN, R. and SMYTHE, L.E., 1979, Lead Burden of Sydney School children, Department of Analytical Chemistry, University of New South Wales.

GIBSON, S.L.M., LAM, C.N., McCRAE, W.M. and GOLDBERG, A., 1967, Archives of Diseases in Childhood, 42, 573.

GOLDBERG, E.D. and GROSS, M.G., 1971, in Man's Impact on Terrestrial and Oceanic Ecosystems (ed Matthews, W.H., Smith, F.E. and Goldberg, E.D.), Massachusetts Institute of Technology Press, Cambridge, p 371.

GREENBERG, M., JACOBZINER, H., McLAUGHLIN, M.C., FUERST, H.T. and PELITTERI, O., 1958, Pediatrics, 22, 756.

GREGORY, R.J., LEHMAN, R.E. and MOHAN, P.J., 1976, in Wegner, G., 1976, op. cit., p 120.

GRIFFIN, T.B., COULSTON, F., WILLS, H., RUSSELL, J.C. and KNELSON, J.H., 1975, Environmental Quality and Safety Supplement, 2, 221.

GRIGGS, R.C., SUNSHINE, I., NEWILL, V.A., NEWTON, B.W., BUCHANAN, S. and RASCH, C.A., 1964, Journal of the American Medical Association, 187, 703.

GUTELIUS, M.F., 1963, Clinical Proceedings of the Childrens' Hospital, Washington, 19, 169.

GUTELIUS, M.F., MILLICAN, F.K., LAYMAN, E.M., COHEN, G.J. and DUBLIN, C.C. 1962, Pediatrics, 29, 1012.

HAENNINEN, H., HERNBERG, S., MANTERE, P., VESANTO, R. and JALKANEN, M., 1978, Journal of Occupational Medicine, 20, 683.

HAMMOND, P.B., O'FLAHERTY, E.J. and GARTSIDE, P.S., 1979, International Conference on Management and Control of Heavy Metals in the Environment, London, September 1979, CEP Consultants Ltd, Edinburgh, p 93.

HARRISON, R.M. and PERRY, R., 1977, Atmospheric Environment, 11, 847.

HARRISON, R.M., PERRY, R. and SLATER, D.H., 1974, Atmospheric Environment, 8, 1187.

HEBEL, J.R., KINCH, D. and ARMSTRONG, E., 1976, British Journal of Preventive and Social Medicine, 30, 170.

HOGBIN, L.E. and BEVAN, M.G., 1976, Transport and Road Research Laboratory Report No. 716, Crowthorne, Berkshire.

HRDINA, K. and WINNEKE, G., 1978, Paper delivered at the Working Conference of the German Association of Hygiene and Microbiology, 2–3 October, Mains.

HURSH, J.B. and SUOMELA, J., 1968, Acta Radiologia 7, 108.

JAMES, A.C. 1977, in Annual Research and Development Report, National Radiological Protection Board, Harwell, Oxfordshire, p 71.

JOSEPHS, D.S., 1977, Public Health (London), 91, 133.

JOST, D. and SARTORIUS, R., 1979, Atmospheric Environment, 13, 1463.

KEHOE, R.A., 1961a, Journal of the Royal Institute of Public Health and Hygiene, 24, 81.

R.A., 1961b, Journal of the Royal Institute of Public Health and 4, 101.

KEHOE, R.A., 1961c, Journal of the Royal Institute of Public Health and Hygiene, 24, 129.

KEHOE, R.A., 1961d, Journal of the Royal Institute of Public Health and Hygiene, 24, 177.

KOTOK, D., 1972, Journal of Pediatrics, 80, 57.

KOTOK, D., KOTOK, R. and HERIOT, J.T., 1977, American Journal of Diseases of Children, 131, 791.

LANDRIGAN, P.J., GELBACH, S.H., ROSENBLUM, B.F., SCHOULTS, J.M., CANDELARIA, R.M., BARTHEL, W.F., LITTLE, J.A., SMREK, A.L., STAEHLING, N.W. and SANDERS, J.F., 1975a. New England Journal of Medicine, 292, 123.

LANDRIGAN, P.J., WHITWORTH, R.H., BALOH, R.W., STAEHLING, N.W., BARTHEL, W.F. and ROSENBLUM, B.F., 1975b. Lancet, i, 708.

LANSDOWN, R.G., SHEPHERD, J., CLAYTON, B.E., DELVES, H.T., GRAHAM, P.J. and TURNER, W.C., 1974. Lancet, i, 538.

LANZKOWSKY, P., 1959, Archives of Diseases in Childhood, 34, 140.

LAWTHER, P.J., COMMINS, B.T., ELLISON, J. McK. and BILES, B., 1973, Commission of the European Communities/United States Environmental Protection Agency: International Symposium on Environmental Health Aspects of Lead, Amsterdam, 2–6 October 1972, Luxembourg, p 373.

LEAD IN FOOD REGULATIONS, 1979, Statutory Instrument No 1254.

LITTLE, P. and WIFFEN, R.D., 1978, Atmospheric Environment, 12, 1331.

LOURIE, R.S., LAYMAN, E.M., MILLICAN, F.K., SOKOLOFF, B. and TAKAHASHI, L.Y., 1958, in The Problems of Addiction and Habituation (ed Hoch, H. and Zubin, J.) Grune and Stratton, New York, p 74.

McINNES, G., 1979, Report No LR 305 (AP), Warren Spring Laboratory, Stevenage, Hertfordshire.

McLEAN, W., 1980, Health Trends, 12, 9.

McNEIL, J.L., PTASNIK, J.A. and CROFT, D.B., 1975, Archives of Industrial Hygiene and Toxicology, 26 (Supplement), 97.

MILLICAN, F.K., LAYMAN, E.M., LOURIE, R.S., TAKAHASHI, L.Y. and DUBLIN, C.C. 1962, Clinical Proceedings of the Children's Hospital, Washington, 18, 207.

MILLICAN, F.K., LOURIE, R.S. and LAYMAN, E.M. 1956. American Journal of Diseases of Children, 91, 144.

MINISTRY OF AGRICULTURE, FISHERIES AND FOOD, 1975, Survey of Lead in Food: First Supplementary Report, HMSO, London.

MONCRIEFF, A.A., KOUMIDES, O.P., CLAYTON, B,E., PATRICK, A.D., RENWICK, A.G.C. and ROBERTS, G.E., 1964, Archives of Diseases in Children, 39, 1.

MOORE, M.R., MEREDITH, P.A., CAMPBELL, B.C., GOLDBERG, A. and POCOCK, S.J., 1977a, Lancet, ii, 661.

MOORE, M.R., MEREDITH, P.A. and GOLDBERG, A., 1977b, Lancet, i, 717.

MORBIDITY and MORTALITY WEEKLY REPORT, 1979, 23, 177.

NEEDLEMAN, H.L., 1977, Studies in Subclinical Lead Exposure, Environmental Health Effects Research Series, Environmental Protection Agency Publication No 600/1–77–037, United States Department of Commerce, National Technical Information Service, Springfield, Virginia.

NEEDLEMAN, H.L., DAVIDSON, I., SEWELL, E.M. and SHAPIRO, I.M., 1974, New England Journal of Medicine, 290, 245.

NEEDLEMAN, H.L., GUNNOE, C., LEVITON, A. and PERESIE, H., 1978, Paper presented to the American Pediatric Society, April 27, New York.

NEEDLEMAN, H.L., GUNNOE, C., LEVITON, A., REED, R., PERESIE, H., MAHER, C. and BARRETT, P., 1979, New England Journal of Medicine, 300, 689.

NEEDLEMAN, H.L. and SHAPIRO, I.M., 1974, Environmental Health Perspectives, 7, 27.

OFFICIAL JOURNAL OF THE EUROPEAN COMMUNITIES, 1977, L. 303, 23.

OFFICIAL JOURNAL OF THE EUROPEAN COMMUNITIES, 1978, L. 197, 19.

PERINO, J. and ERNHART, C.B., 1974, Journal of Learning Disabilities, 7, 26.

PIHL, R.O. and PARKES, M., 1977, Science, 198, 204.

PUESCHEL, S.M., KOPITO, L. and SCHWACHMAN, H., 1972, Journal of the American Medical Association, 222, 462.

RABINOWITZ, M., WETHERILL, G.W. and KOPPLE, J.D., 1974, Environmental Health Perspectives, 7, 145.

RABINOWITZ, M., WETHERILL, G.W. and KOPPLE, J.D., 1976, Journal of Clinical Investigation, 58, 260.

RATCLIFFE, J.M., 1977, British Journal of Preventive and Social Medicine, 31, 258

RICHTER, E.D., YAFFE, Y. and GRUENER, N., 1979, Environmental Research, 20, 87.

ROHBOCK, E., GEORGII, H.W. and MULLER, J., 1980, Atmospheric Environment, 14, 89.

RUMMO, J.H., 1974, Ph D Thesis, University of North Carolina at Chapel Hill.

127

RUMMO, J.H., ROUTH, D.K., RUMMO, N.J. and BROWN, J.F., 1979, Archives of Environmental Health, 34, 120.

RUTTER, M., 1980, Developmental Medicine and Child Neurology, 22, Supplement No 42, 1.

RUTTER, M., GRAHAM, P. and YULE, W., 1970a, A Neuropsychiatric Study in Childhood, Clinics in Developmental Medicine, 35–36, SIMP with Heinemann Medical, London.

RUTTER, M., TIZARD, J. and WHITMORE, K., 1970b, Education, Health and Behaviour, Longmans Green, London.

RUTTER, M. and YULE, W., 1975, Journal of Child Psychology and Psychiatry, 16, 181.

SACHS, H.K., KRALL, V., McCAUGHRAN, D.A., ROZENFELD, I.H., YONGSMITH, N., GROWE, G., LAZAR, B.S., NOVAR, L., O'CONNELL, L. and RAYSON, B., 1978, Journal of Pediatrics, 93, 428.

SACHS, H.K., McCAUGHRAN, D.A., KRALL, V., ROZENFELD, I.H. and YONGSMITH, N., 1979, American Journal of Diseases of Children, 133, 786.

SANDBERG, S.T., RUTTER, M. and TAYLOR, E., 1978, Developmental Medicine and Child Neurology, 20, 279.

SHAPIRO, I.M., NEEDLEMAN, H.L. and TUNCAY, O.C., 1972, Environmental Research, 5, 467.

TANIS, A.L., 1955, American Journal of Diseases of Children, 89, 325.

THOMAS, H.F., ELWOOD, P.C., WELSBY, E. and ST. LEGER, A.S., 1979, Nature, 282, 712.

TURNER, A.C. and CARROLL, J.D., 1980, Report No LR 344 (AP), Warren Spring Laboratory, Stevenage, Hertfordshire.

VOSTAL, J.J., TAVES, E., SAYRE, J.W. and CHARNEY, E., 1974, Environmental Health Perspectives, 7, 91.

WALDRON, H.A., 1979a, Journal of the Royal Society of Medicine, 72, 753.

WALDRON, H.A., 1979b, Lancet, ii, 1070.

WALLER, R.E., COMMINS, B.T. and LAWTHER, P.J., 1965, British Journal of Industrial Medicine, 22, 128.

WARLEY, M.A., BLACKLEDGE, P. and O'GORMAN, P., 1968, British Medical Journal, 1, 117.

WEGNER, G., 1976, Shoshone Lead Health Project (Idaho Department of Health and Welfare).

WHITWORTH, R.H., ROSENBLUM, B.F., DICKERSON, M.S. and BALOH, R.W., 1974, Morbidity and Mortality Weekly Report, 23, 157.

WINDEYER REPORT, 1972, Report of a Committee under the Chairmanship of Sir Brian Windeyer appointed to inquire into Lead Poisonings at the RTZ Smelter at Avonmouth, Cmnd. 5042, HMSO.

YOUROUKOS, S., LYBERATOS, C., PHILIPPIDOU, A., GARDIKAS, C. and TSOMI, A., 1978, Archives of Environmental Health, 33, 297.

ZIEGLER, E.E., EDWARDS, B.B., JENSEN, R.L., MAHAFFEY, K.R. and FOMON, S.J., 1978, Pediatric Research, 12, 29.

Printed in England for Her Majesty's Stationery Office by Oyez Press Limited
Dd 698199   K40   3/80